KU-201-542

Body
for
LIFE

12 Weeks to Mental
and Physical Strength

Bill Phillips
and Michael D'Orso

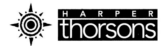
HARPER
thorsons

The Body-*for*-LIFE Program is intended for healthy adults, age 18 and over. This book is solely for informational and educational purposes and is not medical advice. Please consult a medical or health professional before you begin any new exercise, nutrition or supplementation program or if you have any questions about your health. The individuals featured in this book were competing for cash and prizes in an EAS-sponsored shape-up challenge and have received consideration from EAS. They achieved extraordinary results; there are no 'typical' results. Their success stories represent extraordinary examples of what can be accomplished through an integrated system of exercises, nutrition and supplementation. As individuals differ, their results will differ, even when using the same program.

HarperThorsons
An Imprint of HarperCollins*Publishers*
77–85 Fulham Palace Road
Hammersmith, London W6 8JB

The HarperThorsons website address is www.thorsonselement.com

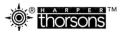

and *HarperThorsons* are trademarks of
HarperCollins*Publishers* Limited

First published by HarperCollins*Publishers*, NY 1999
This edition published by HarperThorsons 2002

11

© 11th Vision, L.L.C. 1999

11th Vision, L.L.C. asserts the moral right to be
identified as the author of this work

A catalogue record of this book is
available from the British Library

ISBN 13 978-0-00-714967-4
ISBN 10 0-00-714967-0

Printed and bound in China by Leo Paper Products

All rights reserved. No part of this publication may be
reproduced, stored in a retrieval system, or transmitted,
in any form or by any means, electronic, mechanical,
photocopying, recording or otherwise, without the prior
written permission of the publishers.

To all the real-life heroes whose paths I have been fortunate enough to cross. Your relentless determination to transform any and all adversity into positive energy and to face the most important challenge of all—*life*—is my inspiration. This book isn't just dedicated to you—it is your creation.

Contents

w.bodyforlife.com   www.bodyforlife.com   www.bodyforlife.com   www.bodyforlife.com   www.bodyforlife.com   www.bodyforlif

Acknowledgments

This book is not the end of anything; it is just the beginning... for you, for me, and for all the men and women who have helped me shape and express the knowledge shared on these pages.

They include, first and foremost, my family—my mother, who has, since day one (literally), been my biggest fan and best friend; my father, who taught me to embrace discipline, order, and learning; my brother, who, growing up, knew just when to kick the tar out of me to keep me in line and still does (albeit not in the front yard but in the gym, where he runs me ragged); my sister, who is, far and away, the true intellectual powerhouse of the offspring; and Ami Cusack, for being there, through so many turning points.

I also wish to express my deep appreciation to: John Elway, whose example has inspired my ascent; Jim Nagle, whose belief in this project helped turn this dream into a realized goal; Dan Sullivan, for being the best Strategic Coach a transforming rugged individualist could ever ask for; and Kal Yee for sharing his wisdom and reference points.

I also thank Leigh Rauen, my all-star word processor, who, through many late nights and early mornings, patiently and skillfully transformed thousands of pages of what looked like ancient Egyptian hieroglyphics into the crisp, clean words you see right here; Sue Daniel-Mosebar and her team of wordsmiths for their attention to detail; Michael Sitzman for his patient perseverance; Brian Harvat and Chris Monck for their dynamic design expertise; my coauthor, Mike D'Orso, who has earned my deepest respect and appreciation for helping me

w.bodyforlife.com   www.bodyforlife.com   www.bodyforlife.com   www.bodyforlife.com   www.bodyforlife.com   www.bodyforlif

harness and forge a lifetime of information into a form that makes sense (at least to him and me); our agent, David Black, who's been successfully converted from a long-time endurance athlete into the Big Apple's budding new pocket Hercules; and our editors—David Hirshey and Jay Papasan—as well as the entire HarperCollins team, including Jane Friedman, whose leadership and understanding opened the door for this book. I'm also extremely grateful for Jeff Stone's vision and courageous spirit; his thoughtfulness and faith will not be forgotten.

This book, like the Program described between its covers, has been a rewarding journey for all of us—a journey that will continue long after these words have been read.

odyforlife.com   www.bodyforlife.com   www.bodyforlife.com   www.bodyforlife.com   www.bodyforlife.com   www.bodyforlife.c

Real-World Proof

"Don't let anybody tell you that you can't do it. You can. It's up to you. Decide to do it and follow through."

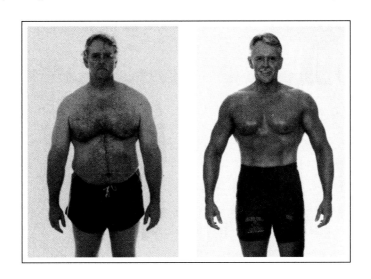

By Porter Freeman

The way I see it, the only difference between a rut and a grave is the depth of the hole. And by the spring of 1996, I had dug myself into a pretty deep hole—eating badly, drinking too many beers, lying on the sofa watching sports on TV instead of participating in them.

w.bodyforlife.com   www.bodyforlife.com   www.bodyforlife.com   www.bodyforlife.com   **www.bodyforlife.com**   www.bodyforlife

I had become a classic couch potato, using different excuses and reasons why I couldn't exercise: a shoulder injury, long hours at work, "I'll start next week," until finally I woke up one day, took a look in the mirror, and realized I was old and fat.

I didn't plan to wrap myself in that huge ball of blubber. It's not something that happened overnight. I didn't just wake up one day and suddenly weigh 260 pounds.

But I *did* suddenly—finally—open my eyes and realize that my body had become something I didn't feel was *me*. What I had let happen to my body was not something I would let happen to my job or to my responsibilities. The neglect, the laziness—that wasn't the way I approached any other aspect of my life. That wasn't who I *was*, not in my heart.

But that's what my body had become—neglected, soft, fat.

It was a friend who helped me get back on track. He gave me a copy of an article Bill Phillips had written and asked me to read it. I took it home and sat down on the side of my bed, with a cold beer and a bag of potato chips. I figured I'd have a little snack, drink my beer, and look through this article before going to sleep.

It was the way Phillips ended that article that nailed me. His words were a direct challenge: *"I've given you every opportunity and every reason to get back in shape. If you don't do it, you might as well go start an ant farm!"*

I swear, it was like he was standing in the room, talking directly to me, saying, "Well, Porter, you've gotten so badly out of shape, I'm going to offer you a shot at hundreds of thousands of dollars' worth of prizes and all the knowledge of how to do it. Are you going to do it? Or are you just going to give up for life?"

I must have read that article three or four times that night, and every time I read it, I got madder and madder. I thought, "Who is he to tell me to go start a friggin' ant farm?" But I soon realized who I was really mad at. I was mad at myself for turning into such a slob. I realized I could no longer go on living like I was. You're not *living* at 260 pounds. You're dying.

bodyforlife.com   www.bodyforlife.com   www.bodyforlife.com   www.bodyforlife.com   www.bodyforlife.com   www.bodyforlife.c

Right then and there, I made a conscious decision to change my life. I was finally fed up with being fed all the time. Just fed, fed, fed.

I became fearless and focused on finishing this challenge. I craved going the entire 12 weeks way more than I craved a piece of key lime pie or a beer. I made up my mind—I was going to make it through those 12 weeks, or they were going to find me dead in the gym.

I really didn't notice a lot of change initially. Other people noticed. And they brought it to my attention. I was so focused on *doing* it that I didn't see all the great things that were happening. A young girl at work walked up to me one day and said, "Porter, your pants are falling off." I hadn't realized that my waist was down to 36 inches, and I was still wearing my old 42-inch pants. That doesn't work.

I can't describe how much inspiration comes from seeing the muscles grow and the fat go. You look in the mirror and it's like meeting an old friend you really liked a lot but haven't seen for quite a while.

I stuck with it, and after 12 weeks, I had lost 54 pounds of body weight and gained much more than just muscle—I had more strength and energy than I'd had in my entire life, and even better than that, I had regained what I knew was my true character.

I'm confident and on track now, but I'll never forget where I once was. I know bad habits wait on us forever. They don't ever go away. They will always be there, just around the corner, lurking and looking for an opening. If you're addicted to food or alcohol or cigarettes or even the wrong person in your life, if you've got a bad habit of any kind, I don't think it just "disappears." If you stop setting goals for your future, if you start living in the moment again, that's when those bad habits will push their way back into your life.

Those 12 weeks—and the months and years that have passed since then—taught me a lesson that I now try to teach to anyone and everyone who will listen:

Anyone can do what I, and thousands of others who have followed the Body-*for*-LIFE Program, have done.

v.bodyforlife.com   www.bodyforlife.com   www.bodyforlife.com   www.bodyforlife.com   www.bodyforlife.com   www.bodyforlife

Don't let anybody tell you that you can't do it. You *can*. It's up to you. Decide to do it, and then follow through on it. I'm telling you, if a 49-year-old guy like me, who works in a bar, who is around almost everything you can think of that is detrimental to good health—if *I* can do it, anyone can do it. Don't wait until you have a heart attack before you remember you have a body!

There are so many people who believe they're too overweight, or too weak, or too old to get in great shape. There are people who think everybody in the gym is in "perfect" condition. That's just not true. Every person in that gym had to start one day, like everybody else. Back early in those 12 weeks, when I got uncomfortable or felt out of place in the gym, I would look in the mirror and tell myself, "You're here because you don't want to look like this any longer." I was much more uncomfortable in that fat body than I was in the gym.

Before those 12 weeks, I would never have thought that I could lay out a red carpet and say to someone, "Come on, be healthy with me." But here I am. I talk with people every day who want to look and feel better. Some of them feel like they're living in hell. They feel like they can't make it another day. But I know, and I tell them, that they can feel as good as I feel. They can make that U-turn. *Everyone* can change his or her body and life with this Program.

I plan to spend the rest of my life helping people get healthy. It's the best feeling I could ever imagine. I'm going to stay in shape for the rest of my life. And, when "that time" comes, I'd like for the Lord to be able to look at me and say, "Gosh, Porter, you look good. You followed the Program, didn't you?"

bodyforlife.com   www.bodyforlife.com   www.bodyforlife.com   www.bodyforlife.com   www.bodyforlife.com   www.bodyforlife.c

The Promise

No matter who you are, no matter what you do,
you absolutely, positively do have the power to change.

What would it take for you to let me help you build your best body ever in as little as 12 weeks?

What if I provided you with a specific exercise and nutrition plan that has been proven to produce startling results for tens of thousands of people from all walks of life—all the way from A-list Hollywood celebrities to world-champion athletes, to moms, merchants, Marines, ministers, and millionaires?

What if I showed you precisely how to make an extraordinary physique transformation by investing *less than 5 percent* of the time available to you each day?

And, what if I promised to be your "Success Coach" for every step of the process—helping you discover your true potential, helping you stay on track, helping you avoid setbacks, and basically doing anything and everything I can to help you achieve your objective of building a better body?

What if I told you that physicians follow my Body-*for*-LIFE Program—to lower cholesterol, to reduce their risk of heart disease, to turn back the hands of time, possibly even to erase years of fitness neglect in a mere 12 weeks?

xv

What if I promised to show you how to attain the body you've always wanted without having to turn your life upside down to get it—without having to spend all your time in a gym doing hours of boring aerobic exercise and starving yourself. I'll even show you how to lose fat while still enjoying your favorite foods, like pizza, pasta, apple pie with ice cream, every week.

Not only that, but imagine waking up in the morning, looking in the mirror, and being downright *excited* about the reflection you see. Imagine *not* having to hide behind baggy sweaters. Imagine your wardrobe made up of clothes that unveil the new you.

Imagine, just 12 weeks from now, having the energy to go all-out from dawn to dusk, having the confidence to do all the things you've been putting off, having the certainty to make the right decision at the right time, knowing you can regain control over *anything* in this world you set your mind to.

Well, you *can*. And it doesn't matter if you're 22 or 62, man or woman, fit or unfit. No matter who you are, this much I promise: You *do* have the power to change.

Ask the men and women whose lives have been changed by the Program described in these pages. They accepted my help, and each and every one of them came out a winner. They emerged from those 12 weeks with a healthier body and an exciting, new life. *They* are the proof—the living, breathing, walking, talking proof—that the Body-*for*-LIFE Program can help you change *your* life, too.

So now are you willing to let me help you?

When you answer "Yes!" to that question, you're not just taking a step, you're making a quantum *leap* toward gaining total control over your body and your life and finally unleashing your true potential in every aspect of your existence.

The process of creating *your* new Body-*for*-LIFE begins the moment you decide to turn the next page.

bodyforlife.com   www.bodyforlife.com   www.bodyforlife.com   www.bodyforlife.com   www.bodyforlife.com   www.bodyforlife.c

Body
for
LIFE

The Breakthrough

Part I

When you gain control of your body,
you will gain control of your LIFE.

A couple of years ago, I attended a fitness convention in Atlanta. It's one of only a few industry trade shows I attend, and therefore, it's one of the only times I come face-to-face with a large number of my readers at once. During the course of that weekend, hundreds of men and women who introduced themselves as avid followers of my magazine came up to shake my hand and chat. What struck me most about the entire experience—what absolutely *floored* me—was how strikingly *out* of shape many of these people were.

Don't get me wrong, I enjoyed meeting *all* these folks, many of whom had been reading my work for years. I even recognized a lot of their names. That weekend I think I met about 600 of my students. Maybe 80 of them looked fit and strong, but the others, who had been receiving the *same* information on exercise and nutrition, looked like . . . well, *like they never had the opportunity to learn about how to get in top shape before.*

On the flight home, I agonized over what I experienced that weekend. I knew then and there that in order to become a better teacher, I had to create a solution that would help these people not just get the facts but *apply* them. I knew I could help these people. I knew it was my responsibility.

1

Anyone who knows me at all or is familiar with me through my writing understands I firmly believe that a strong, healthy mind resides in a strong, healthy body. That, my friends, is a fact. When I see men and women who are out of shape, I see lives not fully lived. I see lost potential. I see people who need someone to help them realize they *can* look and feel better. That's what I see.

You simply cannot escape this reality: Your body is the epicenter of your universe. You go nowhere without it. It is truly the temple of your mind and your soul. If it is sagging, softening, and aging rapidly, other aspects of your life will soon follow suit.

I just don't believe that anyone in this world sets out on a journey to become fat and unhealthy, just as no one decides to become lonely or poor. What happens is, somewhere along the line, slowly and gradually, without even being aware of it, we give up. We give up our values and our dreams one at a time. When people let go of their bodies, it is, quite simply, the beginning of the end.

The night I got home from that trip, I couldn't stop thinking about it. What could I do to help these people *apply* their knowledge? I asked myself that question over and over again. I couldn't sleep. Then, finally, at about 1:15 in the morning, it hit me: They need a *challenge*. A competition. An incentive and the ultimate trophy—my blood-red Lamborghini Diablo.

I recalled how dreaming about someday owning that car helped me back when I was struggling to build my business—it helped me stay focused on my future and lifted my desire when I needed it most. I thought maybe it could do the same for the people I wanted to help—that it could be their *driving force,* too. So, the next day, I put that Lamborghini up as the "Grand Prize" in the most unique self-improvement contest ever.

No one had ever tried issuing a challenge like this before, but something told me I had to do it, even though some people (including my dad, who's also my business advisor) let me know they thought the idea was crazy.

But I experienced something like the voice that whispered to Ray Kinsella in the baseball movie *Field of Dreams*: My instincts told me if I built it, they would come.

bodyforlife.com   www.bodyforlife.com   www.bodyforlife.com   www.bodyforlife.com   www.bodyforlife.com   www.bodyforlife.c

And did they ever…

More than 54,000 people from all walks of life signed up. Cops, cooks, and corporate CEOs. Parents and grandparents (more than a few *great*-grandparents). Men and women who had never lifted a weight in their lives and a few seasoned gym rats who had been trying to build better bodies for years. The entries cascaded in, each individual accepting my challenge.

There were 10 categories, so young and old, men and women alike could all compete and have a chance to win. They were required to take "before and after" photos and write an essay describing their experience and the impact it had on their lives overall. A team of judges, including myself, worked day and night scoring each competitor based on how much they improved their physiques, combined with how well they expressed the experience through their essays.

There—in those essays—was where my expectations and imagination were blown away. I hoped that giving people an incentive and challenging them to *apply* the knowledge I offered them would help them improve their bodies. And it did.

But that's not all. These people were getting physically fit, *and* they were getting their *lives* back in shape. It was, and still is, one of the most enlightening experiences of my life. Accepting this challenge rekindled the flame of desire for tens of thousands, and it broke down walls that were keeping people from moving forward in all areas of their lives.

Many of the men and women who accepted my challenge reported that this Program literally saved their lives. Their risk of heart disease (the number-one killer in America today) was drastically lowered, as well as the risk of being afflicted with other illnesses, such as diabetes, cancer, and osteoporosis.

Beyond even that, the psychological and emotional changes reported by these men and women were (and are) stunning. They described off-the-chart leaps in self-confidence, self-respect, and empowerment. They discovered that taking control of their bodies broke down barriers all around them. People were more attracted to them. They got better jobs. They made greater amounts

w.bodyforlife.com   www.bodyforlife.com   www.bodyforlife.com   www.bodyforlife.com   www.bodyforlife.com   www.bodyforlif

of money. Their relationships with colleagues, family, and friends improved. Their marriages got better. Their sex lives became more satisfying. Old habits that seemed impossible to break suddenly became easy to drop.

And they began to realize that *they really do have the power to help and inspire others* (which, by the way, is, in my opinion, the main reason we're here to begin with). Quite simply, they became more enlightened, more powerful people, in every sense of those words.

During the course of that first challenge, something else unexpected happened: I started getting letters—hundreds of letters—from competitors who no longer *needed* the prizes. They explained that initially my car and the money were the focus, but after a few weeks—as soon as they began being treated differently by others and they began *feeling* differently about themselves—they realized that the biggest and best prize they could win was not anything *I* could give them. (Nope, not even a $200,000 sports car.)

Virtually *all* the people who finished the 12-week challenge felt like winners. After having the opportunity to get to know many of them on a very personal level, I can tell you these real-life champions have done more to inspire me than all the pro athletes and movie stars I know, *combined*. That comment may ruffle some feathers, but it's true.

I could go on and on with literally thousands of examples, but rather than skim the surface of such an incredibly large championship team, I think it would be better to dig in right here with several specific examples.

(By the way, I strongly encourage you to take the time to read these *true* stories *carefully*. These words could change your life. I know because they have already changed mine.)

bodyforlife.com   www.bodyforlife.com   www.bodyforlife.com   www.bodyforlife.com   www.bodyforlife.com   www.bodyforlife.c

He Transformed Tragedy into Triumph

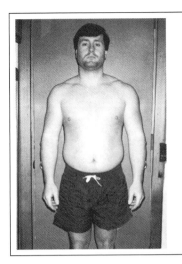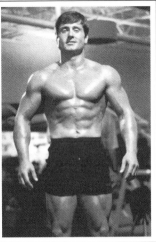

Lynn Lingenfelter's life changed forever on November 11, 1983. He was 16 years old, a starting fullback, and captain of his Pennsylvania high school football team. Along with a friend, he headed into the woods that day near his family's home to hunt small game, something the two had done dozens of times before.

They were climbing a steep mountain slope when Lynn's friend lost his footing. Even before Lynn heard the pop of his companion's .22-caliber rifle, he felt a thump in his back, "As if I'd been slugged with a baseball bat." As he was falling to the ground, Lynn glimpsed back at his friend, who was down on his knees, the weapon still clutched in his hand.

"His eyes were bigger than mine," recalls Lynn.

Lynn actually pulled himself up and tried to run for help. "I went about 30 yards. Then I started to feel really sick. I could see only black and white, and I couldn't hear. I stumbled and fell to the ground. I honestly thought I was going to die. I remember praying and saying, 'God, save me . . . I think I'm going.' Then I must have blacked out."

Almost beside himself with panic and fear, Lynn's friend ran to get help. When he returned, it was with Lynn's younger brother, Mike.

w.bodyforlife.com   www.bodyforlife.com   www.bodyforlife.com   www.bodyforlife.com   www.bodyforlife.com   www.bodyforlif

"They found me lying on the ground, stone cold and blue. I wasn't breathing. By coincidence or fate, Mike had learned CPR in health-education class just a few days earlier. He got me breathing again and held me tight to keep me warm until the paramedics got there and took me to the hospital."

The bullet had entered Lynn's lower back, ripped through his intestines, and come out through the front. He had lost a massive amount of blood while he was lying there on the hill. When he finally got to the hospital, the doctors told his family he had only a fifty-fifty chance of surviving. Lynn had to be given 38 pints of blood to replace what his body had lost.

"I don't remember all that much about the days that followed except I was in a lot of pain. I had one operation after another, one complication after another. I was in the hospital for the better part of five months."

By the time Lynn was finally released, he had lost 50 pounds.

"I couldn't even bench press 100 pounds. But I set a goal of rebuilding my body by the time the next football season started. The doctors said that was *impossible*, which made me even more determined. I trained hard, and my mom fed me well."

When the starting team ran onto the field the first Friday night of that next season, Lynn was among them, once again the starting fullback. The crowd stood and cheered.

"That was one of the most rewarding moments of my life. I remember thinking it was all over now—the tough times my family and I endured because of the hunting accident, those long, long months of not knowing if I'd ever recover. I was ready now for that to become nothing more than a distant memory. Which, as time passed, it did," explained Lynn.

If this were an after-school movie, that would be the end of the story. Music up. Fade out. But Lynn's saga, as he would soon learn, was not nearly over.

"I finished high school, got engaged to my sweetheart, Sara, and enrolled at Penn State University. This was in the fall of 1987. Doctors were being notified at that time of a newly discovered virus that seemed to lead to a fatal disease. One of the means of transmission was through tainted blood. They were

bodyforlife.com   www.bodyforlife.com   www.bodyforlife.com   www.bodyforlife.com   www.bodyforlife.com   www.bodyforlife.c

told that anyone who received blood in recent years should be tested to see if they had the disease. I went in for my test, hardly giving it a second thought. To me, this was a formality, nothing more than that."

Two weeks later, the telephone in Lynn's dorm room rang. (This disease was still new enough at that time that test results were given over the phone.)

"Lynn," the doctor said, pausing for a moment, "you have the HIV virus."

Lynn didn't react. He didn't know *how to* react. A gunshot wound, although horrific, was something he could understand, something he could comprehend. But this . . . beyond what the doctors had told him, he didn't even know what HIV *was*—he only knew it was serious, extremely serious.

"My experience with the shooting had made me believe I could handle anything; I could get out of anything. But I remember all I could think when I got that phone call was, 'How do I get out of *this*?'"

This was a death sentence, or so Lynn was told. The doctors said he had two years to live. Maybe three. Lynn's family was devastated. Breaking the news to his fiancée, Sara, was one of the most difficult things he had ever done.

"Having to tell your fiancée you're dying—that you're HIV-positive—is something I wish no one in the world had to do. We met that evening at her dorm. I remember we were out back, and I said, 'Sara, you're not going to believe this. My test came back positive . . . I have the virus.' It hurt so bad.

"We sat there for hours. She cried so hard she shook from head to toe. We were just kids. Sophomores in college. We had our whole lives ahead of us, so much to look forward to. And in just a few seconds . . . it all melted away."

Sara tried for a time to stay with Lynn, but they believed there was no way it was going to work. Once she left, he dropped out of school.

"I basically dropped out of life. I was in denial, then I was angry, then I hit rock bottom. I was very depressed. I'd sleep 15 hours a day. Sometimes I wouldn't leave the house for a week. I drank beer and ate junk food and watched a lot of TV."

In no time at all, Lynn ballooned to 230 pounds. He tried stemming the tide, but there was no stopping it.

v.bodyforlife.com   www.bodyforlife.com   www.bodyforlife.com   www.bodyforlife.com   **www.bodyforlife.com**   www.bodyforlife

"I'd go to a support group meeting every once in a while, but I wasn't really into it. I knew I needed help, but I didn't really want help. One of the things I've learned is that no one can help you until you've decided you're ready for it."

He also learned that telling people he was HIV-positive meant facing almost certain dread and rejection.

"I remember when one of my friends found out, he asked me to meet him at a restaurant. We talked, and he said, 'My family comes first.' He repeated that phrase four or five times. I wasn't following what he meant. It turned out he didn't want me coming over to his house anymore because he was afraid I would infect his wife and children."

Lynn's response, like so many people in such a situation, was to pull back.

"I learned to just keep my problems to *myself*. I didn't even admit to myself how miserable I was. I can look back now and see what a big mistake that was. One of the first steps in overcoming adversity is to honestly admit how you feel about it, to acknowledge that there is a problem. But I didn't know that then."

And so his downward spiral continued.

"I was sick. I was dying. But I wasn't dying from HIV. I was dying from depression. In a way, I was killing myself. I'd built a prison for myself and filled it with misery. I was so consumed with negative images, I didn't care about myself or anyone around me. It just snowballed. It got out of control. I felt helpless, like I was stuck in the middle of a huge storm, and I couldn't move.

"I knew deep down that I wasn't really a loser. Yet I was losing. I was waiting to die. The doctors told me that's all I had to look forward to. So that's what I was waiting for. I kept waiting. And waiting. Two years went past. Then three. Then *nine*. And I kept waiting."

Lynn wasn't dead. But he wasn't alive either.

"That was a very strange place to be. I began to believe that maybe this HIV was *not* going to kill me. And that forced me to face myself and ask a very tough question:

8

"'*What is the purpose of my life?*'"

It was at this point Lynn began searching for answers. He started having vivid dreams of being a competitive athlete, of being strong and hopeful, with life stretching out in front of him like a bright sunlit path, rather than the dark, hollow tunnel he had been seeing.

"One morning—this was in early '97—I awoke from one of these dreams, went in the bathroom, and looked at myself in the mirror. I looked like crap. I felt like crap. And I told myself I had to change. It was time to take the bull by the horns."

He hauled himself to a local gym and began asking around for information on how to get in shape. One of the guys in the room handed him a copy of one of my publications.

"I had never been so fat. I didn't know what type of nutrition or exercise program I should be following. I looked at this magazine and really liked the way it was written. I felt like someone was talking to me and guiding me.

"I didn't realize it at the time, but what I was finding was a lot more than fitness advice. I could relate to the tone, the language, the attitude of the articles. Beyond information, I was being taught a frame of mind, which inspired me more than all the preachers, teachers, doctors, and counselors who had tried to get through to me before."

Lynn's timing couldn't have been better. One of the issues he picked up that spring included information about my contest. Lynn's competitive fuse was relit.

"It was time for me to show I could be a winner again."

Lynn took everything he had learned about himself, every emotion he had felt, and carried it all into the weight room.

"I couldn't fight the HIV virus physically. I mean, you can't punch it and beat it up. But every time I finished a hard workout, I felt like I had won a battle. Every day I stuck with my nutrition program, I felt I had taken one more step to climb out of the hole I had dug for myself.

"At the end of the first week, I could actually feel a change. I literally felt better about myself. There wasn't much of a *physical* change at that point,

.bodyforlife.com   www.bodyforlife.com   www.bodyforlife.com   www.bodyforlife.com   **www.bodyforlife.com**   www.bodyforlife

but there was a big mental change. I felt good about myself; I'd forgotten what it was like."

Lynn felt—finally—as if his life had direction again.

"Each day I got more and more confident because I was finally moving forward again. I was working toward a goal I could be proud of. Even if I didn't win the contest, I said to myself, 'Worst-case scenario, I'm gonna be in shape at the end of this.' I didn't know if I would win, but I knew I was gonna finish, and that, in itself, would be a victory."

Not only did Lynn's spirit revive, and not only did his body gain shape and strength, but his *health*—his body's response to the disease that lived within it—soared.

"I was—I *am*—HIV-positive. So it was especially important not to deprive my body of nutrients. I had to restrict calories to lose all the fat I put on over the years, so I ate a lot of low-fat, healthy foods like chicken, vegetables, fruit, potatoes, and nutrition shakes.

"It's a bit awkward at first, but after a few weeks, I got used to it, and it wasn't hard to maintain. Today it's just a part of my life. I just wake up and do the right things and make the right decisions throughout the day."

And the rewards?

"When you get in great shape, you have so much more self-esteem. It enables you to handle things better. I'm positive that working out and rebuilding my body helped fight my depression.

"Just knowing I was still capable of accomplishing something gave me confidence. I would come home from the gym each day and look in the mirror and say, 'At least *one* thing in my life is going right.' That was all I needed to keep going.

"This may have saved my life. I've lived more in the past two years than I did in the entire decade before that—a lot more. And I've *learned*. Most of all, I've learned that time lost is lost forever. All those years—my twenties, essentially—they were wasted with frustration and anger, depression and shame.

bodyforlife.com   www.bodyforlife.com   www.bodyforlife.com   www.bodyforlife.com   www.bodyforlife.com   www.bodyforlife.

"For nine years I asked, 'Why *me*?' I replayed that hunting accident again and again in my mind. I obsessed about why my friend didn't have his safety lock on his gun. I wondered how things would have been different if the bullet hit me in the leg instead of going through my gut.

"I was so angry this happened to me. I didn't do anything to anyone. I didn't deserve this. And then, after going through all that, to find out I was HIV-positive . . . it's impossible to understand. It's easy to feel sorry for yourself. It's very hard not to become angry and bitter.

"But I learned that obsessing about it served no purpose other than to torture myself. I've had to forgive everyone and everything—my friend who accidentally shot me, the doctors, the system that let diseased blood be transfused into my body. I had to set myself free from all that and look forward, not back."

It was literally taking his body into his own hands that started to set Lynn free, he told me. All he wanted in the beginning was to improve his body. He had no idea, he says today, that his entire existence would be raised to a greater level of fulfillment and freedom than he has ever known.

"Each day is a gift to me, and I do my best to enjoy it. I smile a lot, which is something I did very little of for nine years. I stay busy. When I was depressed, I used to watch a lot of TV. I think I watched enough TV for the rest of my life, so I try not to do that now. I go on walks with my fiancée, Evey. We go out to dinner. I like to be active. I like to be moving.

"Each day, I try to do something new—to achieve a goal. I recently learned how to in-line skate and surf."

Of all the people I've met in my life, the "new Lynn" may be the most "consistently upbeat" of them all. But why?

"Why am I happy? Because I decided to be happy. That's how simple it is. It's a choice I made. Then I acted on that choice. It took me 10 years to figure out that this was all up to me, and me alone.

"It might sound strange to say that part of making that choice, of deciding to change, is learning how to surrender. I don't mean surrender as in giving up. I mean surrendering the negative emotions that hold so many of us back."

,.bodyforlife.com   www.bodyforlife.com   www.bodyforlife.com   www.bodyforlife.com   www.bodyforlife.com   www.bodyforlife

Blame, shame, resentment. These are the feelings Lynn is talking about. The first step to taking your life into your own hands, he says, is to *open* those hands and empty them of the unhealthy, unproductive things they've been clinging to for so long.

"Complaining makes you more miserable and just makes problems worse. None of the problems I've faced ever went away by complaining. When you complain, you attract other people who complain. That's a dead-end street.

"But it works the other way, too. When you decide to be happy, adventurous, and open-minded, you will find other people who have made the same decision."

Still, there remains the disease. Lynn has been HIV-positive for over 15 years. The virus is there, threatening to take his life at any time—or so some would say.

"I don't look at it that way. I'm not dying; I'm *living*. I'm doing the things I want to do. I'm doing what I can to help other people. I've got a beautiful fiancée who loves me, and I appreciate every day."

Lynn sees the world, and people, in a different way now.

"Because of what I've been through, I've learned to look at other people—*really* look at them. For nine years of my life, I sat on the sidelines and just observed. I watched people. I mean *literally*. Sometimes I'd go to a place like the mall, where I'd sit for hours and just watch people go past.

"And do you know what I saw—what I see? I see most other people dying. Think about it, none of us is going to live forever. We're all here for only a certain amount of time. But how many of us live as if that is true? I think a lot of people need to be taken aside and told, 'Look, you've got only so much more time to live. Make the most of every day, starting *now*—live as you will wish you would have lived when you're dying."

Lynn not only *lives* each day, but he also sets goals, and he dreams.

"My favorite dream now is one where I see myself as an old man. I'm healthy and wise, out on a lake fishing with my grandchildren. The sun is setting, and the gentle summer breeze is getting cool. A storm is coming. Off in

bodyforlife.com   www.bodyforlife.com   www.bodyforlife.com   www.bodyforlife.com   www.bodyforlife.com   www.bodyforlife.

the distance, my wife waves at us, signaling it's time to come back to shore. I ease the boat around. As we head back to the dock, I take the opportunity to tell my grandkids a very valuable lesson their granddad learned the hard way.

"I tell them that sometime during their voyage through life, they're gonna hit a storm. And even though things might get very rough, they should never stop going forward. They must never give up, not even for a moment. If you drop anchor, I tell them, the storm will tear you apart. Look forward, and you will see the beautiful rainbow on the other side. Keep looking forward and move in that direction, and you *will* make it through."

She Lifted Herself Back Up

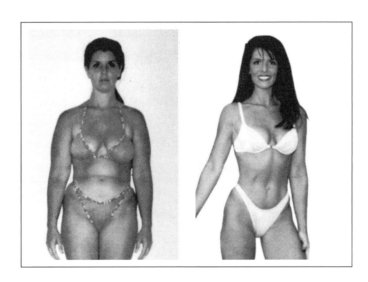

Danielle Coddington, a 33-year-old critical-care nurse and mother of two, from Ft. Lauderdale, Florida, shows that women can experience breakthroughs with this Program as well.

Her story, although not a life-or-death battle like Lynn's, is inspiring—her comeback is one many can relate to. You see, up until a few years ago, Danielle had done a good job of rolling with the punches.

.bodyforlife.com   www.bodyforlife.com   www.bodyforlife.com   www.bodyforlife.com   **www.bodyforlife.com**   www.bodyforlife

Her life, like everyone's, had its share of ups and downs. She had always done a good job of rebounding from setbacks and overcoming obstacles. But after her marriage broke up, she found it difficult to get back on track.

"My life was out of control," explains Danielle. "I knew I needed to do something, but I didn't know what. I was lost."

Fortunately, Danielle's brother recognized that she needed help. He brought her a copy of my video, *Body of Work,* and simply said, "You need to see this."

That night, after putting her kids to bed, she watched the video.

"I couldn't believe what I was seeing—I felt so much *hope*—I connected with the true stories of the real people featured in the movie, and, all of a sudden, I didn't feel alone anymore. I became determined, right then and there, to get control of my body and life, so I accepted Bill's challenge."

Like many others, Danielle's desire was fueled by looking at her before photo.

"I was shocked! I didn't realize how out of shape I was, especially my backside."

Danielle wrote out her goals and got started.

"Within a couple weeks, my body began to change. I could see it. Others could see it. And I felt more optimistic. I couldn't believe how fast my body was changing. In only three months, I lost 21 pounds of fat. Now I'm in better shape than I was in college—I can wear a bikini again and not be embarrassed."

Danielle's success is, in part, due to the support she received from her two children, Rhiannon, seven, and Hunter, five. "They stood by my side all the way and were as excited as I was by the changes. They Rollerblade with me while I run. And when I felt like giving up, they would encourage me to continue. I can't tell you how many times I've heard, 'You can do it, Mommy. Don't quit!' "

Danielle is now inspiring others who have been searching for a way to lose fat and finally get in shape.

"At the hospital where I work, the doctors didn't believe my goals were possible. They had seen photos of others who accepted the challenge, but they

bodyforlife.com   www.bodyforlife.com   www.bodyforlife.com   www.bodyforlife.com   www.bodyforlife.com   www.bodyforlife.

didn't believe the before and after pictures were real, *until* they saw mine. Now they all want to know what I did to achieve such dramatic results. And they're letting me help them.

"When I look back to the moment when I chose to accept Bill's challenge, I see it may have been *the* most important decision of my life. Had my brother not shared the *Body of Work* video with me, I'm not sure where I would be now. I'm not sure if I would have ever lifted myself back up, and I don't even want to think about how that would have affected my children.

"So it's not just that I look better now than I did before, I *feel* better—I'm a *stronger* person, and that's made me a better mother."

Now They're *Loving* Life

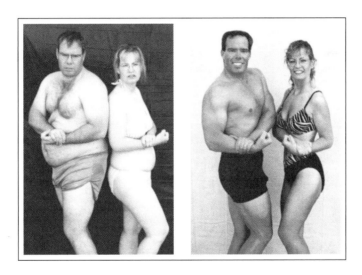

Fred and Renée Scurti, from Parker, Colorado, were doing "okay"—or so they thought. Fred was making a good living as a manager for a computer company, and Renée was working even harder raising their four children. But they, like many other people who have accepted my challenge, were merely *surviving*, rather than *thriving*.

w.bodyforlife.com   www.bodyforlife.com   www.bodyforlife.com   www.bodyforlife.com   **www.bodyforlife.com**   www.bodyforlife

Their wake-up call came one afternoon last fall as Fred was standing in a grocery store checkout line thumbing through magazines. He picked up a copy of my publication and was struck by the before and after stories and photos of men and women who had completed my 12-week Program.

"At first I was skeptical," says Fred. "I couldn't imagine that kind of change happening in as little as 12 weeks. But all those pictures—there must have been 50 or 60 of them—I figured they couldn't be fake. I thought to myself, 'There's gotta be something to this.'"

Fred raced home. Excited to show Renée, he pulled out the magazine and said, "We've got to do this." Renée, too, was awestruck by the transformations. She took one look at Fred and replied, "Let's go for it."

"That decision was one of the most important of our lives. I'd been in bad shape for a long time," explains Fred. "Fifteen years ago, when I was in my early twenties, I was in pretty good condition, but a back injury changed that."

Fred drastically geared back his level of activity. The only exercise he allowed himself was the occasional jog or bike ride. But he kept eating as he always had. Slowly, but surely, year after year, he covered himself with layer upon layer of fat.

"I felt terrible, physically and emotionally. I was constantly depressed. I remember thinking for the first time in my life, maybe I should just accept the fact I wasn't meant to be in good shape. I mean, I was exercising once in a while, eating a low-fat, high-carbohydrate diet, but I kept sinking into worse and worse shape. And I couldn't understand why.

"My kids were getting to the age where they wanted to start doing strenuous things—mountain biking, hiking, soccer—and I couldn't keep up. I was miserable. I knew I could do better as a father, as a husband, as a person."

Renée was in no better condition than her husband.

"As a wife and mother, somebody else's needs were always in front of mine," she says. "I never gave much thought to my own physical well-being."

After accepting the challenge, the couple took pictures of themselves—not an easy thing to put themselves through, as they discovered.

bodyforlife.com   www.bodyforlife.com   www.bodyforlife.com   www.bodyforlife.com   www.bodyforlife.com   www.bodyforlife.c

"I'll never forget the big day we went to pick up those developed pictures," says Renée. "We sat in the car and pulled out the photographs . . . our jaws just dropped. We just . . . well, you just don't *look* at yourself like that . . . not when you look the way we looked. I mean, there we were, in living color. But as painful as looking at those pictures was, it definitely lit a spark and motivated us to get started—now."

With four kids and Fred's full-time job, finding both the time and the place to work out together was a challenge.

"Trying to juggle everyone's schedule—Renée's, the kids', and mine—to work out a way to get to the gym, we just couldn't seem to do that. And there was no question that Renée and I were going to work out *together*. We were in this *together*."

Their solution was to fashion their own "transformation studio" in their basement. "Some free weights, a bench, just the basics," says Fred. Their workout time became the early morning, before the kids woke up, or in the evening, after the kids went to bed around eight o'clock.

"I was concerned that I just wouldn't have the energy to fit this into my life. I was already so tired all the time. But I soon found out that once I got over the initial hump of being very worn out in the very beginning, I had 10 times the energy I ever had before. Getting up an hour early was not a problem at all. As a matter of fact, it happened without even setting an alarm."

"The beauty of doing everything at home," says Renée, "was that we didn't have to depend on anyone else but ourselves. If we failed, it was going to be our fault, and no one else's."

That took care of the exercise side of the program. As for changing their eating habits, it was Fred who had the biggest concerns.

"I thought at first that I was gonna be starving on some kind of diet with this Program. But I soon saw how wrong I was. We went from eating three times a day to eating *six* times a day. We were never hungry. And we were eating *right*. It was wonderful. Right away I thought, 'Wow, I can really do this. I can really stick with this.'"

v.bodyforlife.com   www.bodyforlife.com   www.bodyforlife.com   www.bodyforlife.com   www.bodyforlife.com   www.bodyforlife

"At first, we didn't tell a soul," says Renée. "But after a couple of weeks, we began to see the changes ourselves. We realized this was something we should be sharing with our friends and family.

"And then it kind of snowballed. Everybody we told became involved with our success. They kept checking up on us, and that made it even more important to succeed. We didn't want to let anyone down."

"Commitment," says Fred. "That was one of the main reasons we decided to do this together. I knew if I quit, I was quitting on Renée as well. And I knew that as long as she was in on it, I was in on it, too."

"It starts with being in shape, getting physically fit," says Fred. "But the end result is something totally different, far beyond that. It's how you *feel* about yourself. The level of your confidence."

"I don't mean to sound too melodramatic," explains Renée, "but when you change your life like this, it has a ripple effect on everyone else around you. Because I feel better about myself, my *children* feel better about *themselves*."

"Renée always had confidence and a strong personality," says Fred. "But now she's *more* confident. She's happier, and she radiates that happiness throughout our home. I notice it. The children notice it. It's just changed everything about how we feel as a family.

"Our relationship now is night and day from what it was before. We've been married for 15 years, but we've never done anything like this before. Together we lost 98 pounds of fat (Fred lost 57 and Renée lost 41) in just over three months, and we gained muscle tone, strength, and energy.

"We accomplished this goal as a *team*, and that's been wonderful for our relationship," explain Fred and Renée.

"We were doing fine before this. We didn't have any great problems. But I can see now that we were just living life; now we're *loving* life."

bodyforlife.com   www.bodyforlife.com   www.bodyforlife.com   www.bodyforlife.com   www.bodyforlife.com   www.bodyforlife.c

The End of the Beginning

When that first contest was over—I was awestruck by how many great people there are in this world who *don't even know they're great*. They've been convinced they don't deserve to look and feel better. So they've given up.

Once I became aware of how widespread this problem was, I realized my work had just begun—that "voice" told me I had to do even more. I had to share this experience with everyone I could, allowing others to see what kind of change is possible for them, too.

First, I decided I would make a documentary movie, *Body of Work*, to spread the word. The movie is a celebration of what is best about the human spirit. It's about the growth and goodness we go through when we, with all our inner strength, embrace and overcome those challenges.

Body of Work has been seen by more than two million people . . . and counting. I offer it free on video to anyone—*anyone*—who agrees to make a $15 donation to the Make-A-Wish Foundation® *if* after watching the movie they feel that they received something of value—if they were inspired or enlightened. The amount of these donations is currently over $1,250,000 and continues to climb every day. (By the way, it would be my pleasure to send *you* a free *Body of Work* video, too. If you're interested, call 1-800-297-9776 [Dept. #24] or visit our website at www.bodyforlife.com.)

The movie has inspired even more people to accept my challenge to apply the Body-*for*-LIFE Program and allow it to help them rebuild their bodies and strengthen their lives. More than 200,000 men and women—nearly four times the first year's total—entered last year. It looks like this year's total should pass, believe it or not, *one million*.

I'm determined to help *each* and *every* one of these people experience the kind of breakthrough Lynn, Danielle, Fred and Renée, and so many others have achieved. As you'll discover, *that's* the purpose of *this* book—to help you learn precisely how to become our next real-life success story, in as little as 12 weeks.

w.bodyforlife.com   www.bodyforlife.com   www.bodyforlife.com   www.bodyforlife.com   www.bodyforlife.com   www.bodyforlife

Crossing the Abyss

———————— Part II ————————

There is a world of difference between
knowing what to do and actually doing it.

I consider it a privilege when people let me help them. I love it when they succeed. But as numerous as the success stories are, I'm repeatedly reminded of the fact that there are still millions of people who have yet to discover their true potential.

Many of them know how to exercise. Some know how to eat right, too. In fact, this vast and ever-expanding population of people who have yet to successfully change even includes doctors and professors who know all about the human body.

What these people are missing is the ability to *apply* knowledge. Without that skill, it doesn't matter how much you know, you'll be stranded at the edge of an infinite chasm I call *the abyss*.

Until you discover how to cross the abyss, you will struggle. You will have setbacks. And you may even lose hope.

However, those who do cross the abyss—those who know *and* do—enjoy not only tremendous changes in the way they look and feel—they move forward, fast, in all areas of their lives.

So how do you take that leap and join those on the other side who are now *thriving*, not merely *surviving*? Well, that's what I'm about to share with you.

v.bodyforlife.com   www.bodyforlife.com   www.bodyforlife.com   www.bodyforlife.com   **www.bodyforlife.com**   www.bodyforlif

But before I do, we need to have a little "heart-to-heart talk." You see, as you may have already noticed, this book is about much more than physical fitness—it's about *life*.

I've discovered that any discussion of the correct way to get in shape and stay in shape is, in actuality, a discussion of how you've lived your life up to this point and how you will live it in the future.

Therefore, to help you make the dramatic changes in your body and life, which you *do* have the potential to make, I'm going to have to ask you some very personal questions throughout this section. And you're going to have to look inside—*deep inside*—for the honest answers. This, in and of itself, is a challenge, but it is vitally important.

You see, the dramatic transformations, like the ones you read about in the last section, started with honest reflection, not with merely buying some home-exercise gadget, nor stocking up on the latest "miracle pill." Superficial approaches like that *never* truly work.

Real change always starts on the inside. And that is where you're going to have to find the answer to the first question:

Have you made the decision to change?

Most people I ask tell me they've made this decision. But how many people have truly decided to change? Very few. Why? Because there's a big difference between deciding something and having *reasons* to actually do it.

When you make a decision to make a change *and* you know your reasons, you will harness the force—the desire to make something happen. So now I ask:

What are your reasons for making the decision to change?

You see, it's one thing to *say* you've decided to lose 30 pounds of fat and get in shape. It's a whole other thing to have your doctor tell you you'll be dead in a year and never see your children's children if you don't lose 30 pounds, pronto.

I know that you know deep down inside you have a number of reasons for deciding to change. I can't tell you exactly what they are, but I can tell you they are there.

bodyforlife.com   www.bodyforlife.com   www.bodyforlife.com   www.bodyforlife.com   www.bodyforlife.com   www.bodyforlife.

Here's a question that will begin to help you find *your* reasons:

When you look at yourself, do you honestly like what you see?

It's important to *really* look. Since we all "see" ourselves every day, we often don't notice if we're slipping. If we're not careful, before long, the image we have of ourselves in our minds will not be in sync with reality.

I suggest you also have someone take a photo of you, standing relatively relaxed with your arms at your sides, in a pair of shorts or a swimsuit. Get that photo developed and *look* at it.

Here are a few more questions that will help you identify *your* reasons:

How do you feel deep down inside?

How do you really feel about yourself?

Are you confident, energetic, and strong?

Do you often wonder if you're on the right path?

What are the pros and cons of continuing in the direction you're going?

Would you like to create a brighter future?

When you answer these questions, your reasons for making the decision to change will become clear. When they do, write them down on a piece of paper, and read what you've written first thing in the morning and again at night before you go to sleep. Do this every day throughout your 12-week Program. These reasons will remain your guiding light, your beacon, during the journey you have now *decided* to begin.

Focusing Your Future Vision

Once you've identified your reasons for making the decision to change, the next question I need you to answer is this:

What are the five most important, specific accomplishments you need to make, within the next 12 weeks, for you to be pleased with the progress of your body and life?

Please take just a few minutes to think this one through, then continue.

.bodyforlife.com   www.bodyforlife.com   www.bodyforlife.com   www.bodyforlife.com   **www.bodyforlife.com**   www.bodyforlife

If you found it easy to identify five *specific* things you know have to occur between today and 12 weeks from now for you to be pleased with the progress of your body and life, that's a good sign. It means you're looking forward and that you have what I call *future vision*.

If you struggled a bit—if you couldn't quickly identify five specific accomplishments but you at least identified two or three you were certain of, then you're doing pretty good, but there's room for improvement.

Now, if you found it extremely difficult to come up with any specific answers to this question—if it caught you completely off guard—you are not alone.

The truth is, most people have a very hard time answering this seemingly simple question. It's just not something most people focus on. However, because we want to change—because we want to move forward—we need to make sure we're *looking forward*.

In other words, we need to focus on our future vision.

Let me explain. We all have three types of vision—historical, present, and future. Where you are in life and where you will go from here has a lot to do with what type of vision you allow to dominate your thoughts, decisions, and actions.

A person whose actions are dominated by historical vision believes that just about everything that's important, enjoyable, or significant in his or her life has already happened.

These folks spend a lot of time reflecting on *the good old days*—talking about high school parties, prom night, the fumble they recovered in the big football game, how they used to be in great shape. *Used to be.* That's the mantra of people with historical vision. It's as if their lives are over. They would rather look backward than forward because it's easier to reminisce about where they've been than to try to figure out where they're going. People with that kind of focus are reluctant to accept new ideas or opportunities, and they have trouble sticking with anything challenging.

What's worse is that individuals with historical vision are very uncomfortable with the growth of others because it threatens the structure and apparent

bodyforlife.com   www.bodyforlife.com   www.bodyforlife.com   www.bodyforlife.com   www.bodyforlife.com   www.bodyforlife.

equilibrium of their own lives. They are uncomfortable with evolution, so a positive change in those around them (husband, wife, friends) is something they fear. The fact is they probably feel, at some level, that they're going to be left behind if they don't start moving their own behinds. And the truth is, they're probably right.

The fact that your eyes are looking at these words on this page right now, and you and I are sharing this learning experience—a learning experience about how to create a better future—makes it very unlikely your thoughts are dominated by historical vision. (If you were a past-based thinker, you'd probably be watching reruns of *Gilligan's Island* or whatever's on the boob tube at this moment, instead of putting forth a focused effort to grow and learn.)

However, I've discovered that far too many people who want to create a better body and more fulfilling life are dominated by what I call present vision. They aren't obsessed with going back in time, but neither are they focused nearly enough on the future. These people have tremendous potential to improve, rapidly. They just need guidance—someone to help them look forward instead of focusing so much on this moment.

People whose daily actions are governed by future vision are, on the other hand, continually growing. They are constantly taking on new and bigger challenges. They're always creating, modifying, and improving their vision of the future. What has happened to such people in the past is not ignored or denied—those experiences are used to develop skills that help them get where they want to go. But it's *always* where they're going that remains the primary focus.

When you develop a strong future vision, you don't have to force yourself to set goals, your mind just compels you to set them. And every time you accomplish an objective, it's not the end of anything; it's the beginning, the starting point for another stage of an ongoing journey of progress, development, growth, and adventure.

Which brings us back to your response to my last question. If you could not quickly and decisively identify five specific things which you need to

.bodyforlife.com   www.bodyforlife.com   www.bodyforlife.com   www.bodyforlife.com   www.bodyforlife.com   www.bodyforlife

accomplish within the next 12 weeks for you to be pleased with your progress in life, now is the time to focus your future vision by answering this question:

What changes in your body and life do you wish you could create within the next 12 weeks?

Take a few minutes to think it over. Be open, honest, and spontaneous. Please do not be concerned about what other people might want you to want.

The things which come to your mind quickly—the things that conjure up powerful emotions and get you as excited about your future as a kid is on Christmas morning are your *dreams*. When you imagine them actually happening, you'll feel the energy.

Now, I need you to take the five most exciting things you come up with and turn them into powerful, specific statements. I need you to write them down. For example, if you thought "gain muscle" and "lose fat," you might write the following sentences: "Within 12 weeks, I will gain 10 pounds of muscle." And "Within 12 weeks, I will lose 20 pounds of fat."

By composing sentences like these—by defining and stating your wish—and by setting a deadline (within 12 weeks), you'll be transforming your dreams into *goals*. You'll be taking a big step toward making them happen. These dreams are no longer lodged somewhere deep in the shadows of your subconscious mind. They're now being pulled out into the light of day. They're now things you are very consciously aware of. You know what? Now that you dug 'em up, you can't put 'em back. You're going to think about these things all the time. And that's good. You *should* think about them because that's part of the process of making your dreams come true.

However, you must transform your dreams into goals and *write them down*. It really does work. Here's proof: Back in 1953, a Harvard University study showed that three percent of the students graduating that year actually wrote down their specific career goals. Twenty years later, a team of researchers interviewed the class of '53 and found that the three percent who had written down their goals were worth more financially than the other 97 percent combined.

bodyforlife.com   www.bodyforlife.com   www.bodyforlife.com   www.bodyforlife.com   www.bodyforlife.com   www.bodyforlife

It's very important to understand the difference between dreams and goals. Dreams are things you wish for—things you enjoy thinking about but really don't know when or if they'll happen. Goals, on the other hand, are specific things you have decided you need to accomplish within a clearly defined period of time. For example, "Someday I'm going to get in great shape" is a dream. "Within 12 weeks, I will lose 20 pounds of fat" is a goal.

Here's another important point: Your goals come from your dreams. (I'll bet you didn't realize that, did you?) Powerful dreams of positive changes in your life add even more fuel to your transformation. But you must create goals that are in sync with your dreams in order to move forward in your life and feel good about yourself, your progress, and your future potential.

Something else, while we're on the subject: When you accomplish a goal, it helps your dreams become even more inspiring, which, in turn, creates even more goals and more desire. When you begin the process of setting and achieving goals, you'll immediately begin creating grander dreams. And that creates optimism, which feels pretty darn good in case you've forgotten. When you're optimistic, you can't help but focus on the future. It's just so exciting, you can't wait to get there.

Are you starting to see how all that works? Can you see that when you don't set and achieve specific goals, you can't create greater dreams, and when you stop dreaming, you don't have anything to look forward to, so you don't look forward, you look down, or back?

You should set goals that are ambitious yet attainable. You might not know where the limit is, especially if you're getting into an area where you don't have a lot of experience or knowledge. So here's a tip on how to set your goals: Find an example—someone who has accomplished what you want to accomplish—and set your goals based on that. If you want to lose fat and get in great shape (notice it's still a dream—no specifics or deadline yet), find someone who was in your present condition, or thereabouts, and take a look at what he or she was able to achieve. You might find an example (a role model, as some call it) who lost 21 pounds of fat in 12 weeks. Okay, there's your goal. It's a

.bodyforlife.com   www.bodyforlife.com   www.bodyforlife.com   www.bodyforlife.com   www.bodyforlife.com   www.bodyforlife

great place to start because that person is living proof it can be done. (Of course, you can look at what others have accomplished to help you set goals in all areas of your life.)

Once you create your list of goals, don't just put it away and never look at it again. Hang on to it and read it first thing in the morning when you get up and again at night before you go to sleep, every day. Try reciting each statement aloud as if you were describing your own future to someone else. Speak with total confidence and assurance.

Practice eliminating doubt from your tone of voice. And don't describe your future success as something you "hope" to achieve. Picture it as something you absolutely will accomplish. You see, hope is not a strong enough emotion to create the desire you'll need to keep you going. You must be convinced that what your imagination has created is your future reality.

In addition to reading your goals first thing in the morning and again at night, focus on your future vision throughout the day as well. For example, if you're doing 20 minutes of aerobic exercise on a stationary bike (which bores me silly, so I have to focus on something else), use that time to focus on your future vision. Rather than "zoning out" or thinking about how much fun you had at that party last Saturday, think about the exciting journey you are embarking upon.

Maybe you need an actual image of your new self to help you focus. Find one—a photo in a magazine, perhaps a before and after photo of someone who has made the type of transformation you would like to make. Cut it out and focus on that image first thing in the morning and again at night.

After you look at that image, close your eyes for just a few minutes. See yourself with a strong, lean body; your posture is good—shoulders back, chest out, chin up—a look of confidence, control, and satisfaction on your face.

Think about how proud you will feel when you look at yourself and see the result of your efforts. Forget about everything else for a few minutes—think only of your future vision. Feel your physique taking shape.

Imagine other people seeing you with your new body. See them seeing you. Listen to what they're saying. Feel the surge of energy and pride.

bodyforlife.com   www.bodyforlife.com   www.bodyforlife.com   www.bodyforlife.com   www.bodyforlife.com   www.bodyforlife.

With practice, you'll eventually become so good at this that it will be like watching a movie. You'll see everything with exhilarating clarity.

Remember that everything you do in the real world is merely an external manifestation of what has already happened in your mind. That's where the relatively well-known maxim, "If your mind can conceive it, you can achieve it" comes from. And it's true. In your mind, anything is possible. Anything you want to happen in your life—that you really want to achieve—you have to rehearse in your mind.

You see, when we're born, our minds have few limitations. They work unfailingly for us. We're not born with all this fear and doubt. Those things are learned. We learn what we can't do, what we're *not* capable of. When we were kids, we believed anything was possible. Limitations, impossibilities—these are things our minds become programmed to believe.

But now you know you can change. By teaching yourself to believe in your future vision, you are positioning and preparing yourself to move onward and upward—to ascend. And soon when things don't go your way, you'll be able to pick yourself up because your future vision will be stronger than your setbacks, and it will pull you right back on track. Doing the particular things you need to do to move toward that future vision will feel right, and you will enjoy the comforting, assuring feeling that whatever happens will happen, but in the end, you will get where you want, need, and deserve to go.

Transforming Patterns of Action

Patterns of action are like habits. They are the "rules" we follow *automatically*—the things we do that we don't even think about. We've all got them. We have patterns of action for how we work, how we eat, how we relate to other people, how we do just about everything. What makes a pattern of action good or bad is simply whether it takes us closer to or pushes us further away from our goals.

.bodyforlife.com   www.bodyforlife.com   www.bodyforlife.com   www.bodyforlife.com   www.bodyforlife.com   www.bodyforlife

Now that we've decided to change and we've become more clear about our future, we need to look at our patterns of action, which brings us to the next important question I need you to answer:

Which three patterns of action might prevent you from reaching your goals?

For example, if someone's goal is to lose 20 pounds of fat, he would need to stop eating low-nutrient, high-calorie foods. Another pattern of action he might need to get rid of is skipping workouts. You see, these habits will prevent progress, so they have to go—they are what I call "unauthorized."

Think about it and write down the three patterns of action which you believe might hold you back. Once you've done that, please answer this question:

Which three new patterns do you need to establish to reach your goals?

For example, if someone's goals include gaining 10 pounds of muscle, he would need to get in the habit of regularly lifting weights. He might need to start eating more often and getting more sleep.

You must identify both the patterns you will stop and the new ones you will start. You see, I've discovered one of the reasons so many people fail to break their bad habits is because they merely focus on what they *shouldn't* be doing—what they *shouldn't* eat, that they *shouldn't* smoke or drink—all these things they *shouldn't* do.

I recommend you focus just as much on things you should start doing because new patterns help "crowd out" the unauthorized ones.

By the time you've identified three patterns of action that are unauthorized and three *new* ones you need to start, you'll be on your way. And, even though it might have taken you years to develop the patterns of action that brought you to this point in your life, it's not going to take you anywhere near that long to change them; in fact, it takes less than four weeks before these new patterns of action will feel more natural to do than to not do. Then you will be able to *apply* the knowledge which you are about to learn.

bodyforlife.com   www.bodyforlife.com   www.bodyforlife.com   www.bodyforlife.com   www.bodyforlife.com   www.bodyforlife.

Overview of How to Cross the Abyss

- Make the decision to change.

- Identify *your* reasons to change and write them down.

- Focus on your future vision.

- Dream of what you would like to achieve within 12 weeks.

- Transform five of those dreams into goals by giving them a deadline, a way to measure them, and writing them down.

- Identify three unauthorized patterns of action that may hold you back and write them down.

- Identify three new patterns of action that will help you reach your goals and write them down.

- Read what you've written first thing in the morning and again at night each and every day of your 12-week Program.

v.bodyforlife.com   www.bodyforlife.com   www.bodyforlife.com   www.bodyforlife.com   **www.bodyforlife.com**   www.bodyforlife

Separating Myth from Fact

———————— Part III ————————

Once the truth is revealed,
the path becomes clear.

Now you've reached the point where you're ready to move forward. You've done a great deal of thinking so far. You've answered questions most people never even ask. And you've learned how to cross the abyss.

At this point, we've just gotta "eat right and exercise."

Eat right and exercise.

It's really quite simple, don't you think?

What's that? You don't *get it*?

Oh, c'mon, what could be more elementary than "eat right and exercise"?

If it were that simple, why is it that if you ask 100 different "experts," you'll get 100 different answers? On top of that, you've got those TV infomercials that claim this or that exercise gadget or miracle pill is *the* answer. All those workout videos, dozens of fitness magazines, and hundreds of books.

So we've got a lot of answers. That's great, *right*?

Well, no. What we have *really* got is a junk heap of false conclusions, endless contradictions, and half-baked exercise and nutrition theories that are creating so much uncertainty and confusion, most people don't know which way to turn.

w.bodyforlife.com   www.bodyforlife.com   www.bodyforlife.com   www.bodyforlife.com   **www.bodyforlife.com**   www.bodyforlife

Before you can begin your 12-week transformation, you need to clear your mind—try to forget everything you've heard about how to eat right and exercise. (It's a lot easier to paint a picture on a blank canvas than it is to paint over someone else's mess.) But some folks have a hard time truly clearing their minds.

You see, some of these myths have been lurking around for so long they have just been accepted as truth. Unless they're eliminated, they rear their ugly heads when you least expect them and threaten to destroy your efforts to build a stronger, leaner, more energetic body.

Let's not allow that to happen—let's conquer these myths—let's separate fact from fiction and create some clarity, right here, right now, once and for all.

Myth: Aerobics is better for shaping up than weight training.
Fact: To transform your physique, you *must* train with weights.

Walking around the block or simply climbing a flight of stairs is better than just sitting there doing nothing. But the best form of exercise, for reshaping your body, is weight training.

Through resistance training, you can also significantly increase your metabolic rate—the rate at which your body burns fat. As you may already know, when you gain muscle, your body requires more energy to maintain that new muscle. Fat weight doesn't require any energy at all to maintain—it just sits there. That's why weight training is even superior to aerobic exercise for people who want to lose fat: It addresses the core of the problem—the rate at which your body uses energy.

If you do nothing but aerobic exercise, even if you eat less, your results will not be optimal. Yes, you may lose weight. But your overall shape will stay the same. If you start an aerobic exercise program shaped like a pear, the most likely result is you will wind up looking like a smaller pear—which is fine, if that's what you want. But that's not what I call a transformation.

With weight training, you not only burn fat but you can also change the shape of your body—you can build wider shoulders, so your waist looks more

bodyforlife.com   www.bodyforlife.com   www.bodyforlife.com   www.bodyforlife.com   www.bodyforlife.com   www.bodyforlife.c

narrow. You can build muscular arms; lean, defined abdominal muscles; strong legs; and you become empowered, confident, and strong.

So even though aerobic exercise does help burn fat, when it comes to transforming your body, proper weight training can't be beat.

Myth: If you exercise, it doesn't matter what you eat.
Fact: If you exercise, it matters *even more* what you eat.

More Americans are exercising now than ever before. And that's got to be good news, right? We must be making up for those high-fat, high-calorie diets with the positive effects of exercise because those effects are just, well, so positive.

Think again. Despite the fact that more and more people are giving exercise a try, we're still seeing a rapid increase in the number of Americans who are obese and who are suffering from health problems caused by being very "unfit."

In fact, there are in excess of 58 million clinically obese men and women in America today, and we spent more than $100 billion last year alone to treat diseases such as cancer, diabetes, stroke, heart disease, and other ailments that are caused, more often than not, by a lack of "fitness."

What I see are literally millions of people who are completely overlooking the fact that physically active individuals need more nutrients than their sedentary counterparts. So many people are so misinformed about this topic. I wish I could go to every fitness center in North America and tell every single person who's exercising—whether they're walking or running, swimming or spinning, lifting weights or whatever—that without optimal levels of the nutrients your body needs, you are not going to get the results you're looking for. If you're anything like me, you exercise to create a positive result, not because you've got nothing else to do. In fact, you may be doing more harm than good because when you exercise a nutrient-deficient body, you're not making it healthier: You're actually creating a worse nutrient deficiency.

.bodyforlife.com   www.bodyforlife.com   www.bodyforlife.com   www.bodyforlife.com   www.bodyforlife.com   www.bodyforlife

Believe me, folks, I've tested this thing every way to Sunday. I know thousands of people, many of whom are probably just like you, who had all but given up on ever discovering how to successfully transform their physiques. Many of them had the technical information on nutrition and exercise but couldn't cross that abyss we talked about earlier. Others had a reason, they set a goal, and they were prepared to cross the abyss, but they didn't have the correct information—they had misinformation. In every case, something was missing, and the person was left believing that "Exercise only works for people with the right genetics," or "There's something wrong with my system," or "I must have a thyroid hormone problem or something."

I mean, let's face it. If we give something a solid effort, if we really put our hearts and souls into it, not just once but time and time again, and it still doesn't work, eventually we're going to get frustrated and give up. Working hard and going nowhere is unrewarding and dispiriting. It's downright frustrating.

The bottom line is this: If you don't have the nutrients in your system to recover, much less improve, following intense exercise, it's like you're flicking a lighter with no butane—you might get a spark but no flame. You have to have both—the fuel and the spark. You have to have the material for that fire to burn, and you have to have the spark to create the flame.

Essentially, there are a bunch of people out there with blistered thumbs just slapping away at a lighter and burning out the flint because there's no fuel in their bodies to create combustion. The result, naturally, is frustration. Imagine if you were holding a lighter and you just sat there going *flick, flick, flick, flick*—and nothing happened.

Eventually you'd say, "Screw this. This lighter doesn't work." And you'd throw the thing away. Well, this is what too many people do with the idea of exercise. They give it a go, without feeding themselves properly, and then they quit in despair.

However, it doesn't have to be that way. By not becoming a victim of the myth that exercise alone is all you need to get fit—by accepting the fact that

bodyforlife.com   www.bodyforlife.com   www.bodyforlife.com   www.bodyforlife.com   www.bodyforlife.com   www.bodyforlife.

optimal nutrition is just as important as exercise—you will be one step closer to achieving the level of success you rightfully deserve.

Myth: If women lift weights, they'll get "bulky."
Fact: Resistance exercise helps women create lean, toned bodies.

The number of women using free weights in America has more than doubled in the past 10 years, from less than eight million in 1988 to more than 17 million in 1997. Almost half the competitors who have successfully completed my 1999 Transformation Challenge are women—that's up from 5 percent the first year and 20 percent the second. And let me tell you, their transformations are spectacular! Very often, they *completely* change the shape of their bodies.

That's partially because fat takes up five times as much space as muscle. This means if you replace the fat on your hips or thighs with the same weight in muscle, your thighs will get much smaller.

Women worried about "bulking up" with weights need to understand this. It's your body composition that determines how you look. By replacing fat with muscle, you can make an astounding transformation without feeling weak and unhealthy. Women should actually be concerned about not having enough muscle, rather than too much.

Myth: Weight training is only for young athletes.
Fact: People of all ages should be weight training.

If we don't work out, we lose muscle mass as we grow older. And, believe it or not, this process begins kicking in at about age 25! This is when most men and women start seeing their body-fat levels increase. From his early thirties to his mid-sixties, the average American man's body-fat level often doubles, from about 18 percent to 36 percent. In that same time frame, the average American woman's body fat can bulge from 33 percent to 44 percent.

Okay. We get older, we get fatter. We get fatter, we lose muscle mass. We lose

Separating Myth from Fact

37

muscle mass, we lose strength. We lose strength, and we do indeed become fragile, weak, and prone to a host of physical disabilities.

But this is not inevitable. Recent university studies show that weight training makes a significant contribution to the quality of life of anyone, even—and often, especially—those in their potential golden years. A study at Tufts University showed that among a group of men between 60 and 72 years old, a three-day-a-week weight-training program caused an average increase in flexibility and strength of up to 200 percent. (So much for the nonsense about weight training making you "muscle-bound." Studies like this show quite the opposite—that the proper use of free weights increases the body's strength and flexibility.)

Fortunately, aging baby boomers are starting to catch on. Statistics show that the largest recent surges in exercising, including weight training, among the American population is by men and women over the age of 50.

The fact of the matter is, you don't have to have some type of advanced level of fitness or some special skill before you can begin training with weights. You don't have to go through some type of special conditioning before you step into a weight room. No matter what your current level of fitness is—whether you're a beginner or you've been working out for years—if you're healthy, you are ready to step into the weight room right now.

Myth: The longer you exercise, the better.
Fact: Too much exercise *prevents* results.

This myth is one I battle *daily*. The workouts I recommend are brief, intense, and highly effective. They stimulate the muscles and burn fat. And they take less than four hours a week. That's it. That's all you need. And despite what so many people believe, working out more is not better. It's really not.

I've learned from countless hours of scientific research, personal experience, and most importantly, from thousands of people in the real world that working out *too* much actually takes us further away from our goals.

bodyforlife.com   www.bodyforlife.com   www.bodyforlife.com   www.bodyforlife.com   www.bodyforlife.com   www.bodyforlife.c

Not only is it hard on the body but it is also very draining on the mind. Brief, intense periods of exercise produce impressive physical results while actually clearing the mind, relieving stress, and allowing us to focus on accomplishing the day's goals. (That sounds good, doesn't it?)

Your workouts should provide the *precise* amount of stimulation needed to trigger an adaptation response. You work out with weights only three days a week and do a special kind of aerobic training three days a week on alternating days. No more. No less. Once you stimulate the muscle, you need to move on and start the recovery process because that is where the magic happens. (I'll explain that "magic" in a minute.)

With exercise, as with so many things, it's not as simple as "the more you put in, the more you get back." There is a point of diminishing returns beyond which, if you keep pushing your body, it will begin working against you.

I've found most people who work out a lot and have little to show for it rarely think working out less could produce better results faster. Instead, they work out longer and more often, clearly under the false assumption that more is better. (Please don't make this mistake!)

Myth: Muscles grow while you're working out.
Fact: Muscles grow while you're resting and recuperating.

As I alluded to earlier, an intense weight-training workout is just the spark—the real magic happens later, not while you're working out but while you're resting. With that in mind, let's take a closer look at what we really want to happen during a weight-training workout.

During the workout, we're trying to slightly damage the muscle fibers by overloading them. I don't want to get into a bunch of complicated anatomy and such, but when you work out with free weights properly, you cause micro-trauma to the targeted muscle tissue. Once that occurs, the body responds by mobilizing its muscle-rebuilding workforce.

Imagine a muscle cell as a structure, a building. And imagine exercise as a

.bodyforlife.com   www.bodyforlife.com   www.bodyforlife.com   www.bodyforlife.com   www.bodyforlife.com   www.bodyforlife

slight earthquake. After the tremor causes structural damage to the building, a repair team has to come in and rebuild it.

This is essentially what happens after an effective free-weight workout. You slightly damage muscle cells; then your body mobilizes to fix that damage. This repair work requires energy that, under the right circumstances, will be pulled from your stored body fat. That's another reason effective weight training will help you burn fat. You'll actually tap into the energy sitting dormant in fat and use it to fuel the growth of muscle when you follow this Program.

There's more to this, of course, including the importance of nutrients which are probably not going to be found in that stored body fat—nutrients such as amino acids (which come from quality protein), vitamins, minerals, creatine, and other essential raw materials needed to build a better body.

I cannot emphasize enough how important it is to give your muscles time for this process to go full circle. If you work out again before the muscles have had time to rebuild, you will short-circuit the recovery process. And that's *not* good.

Let's go back to that earthquake analogy one more time. Imagine if that rebuilding workforce were in the process of putting that house back together—they were almost done with their repair work when, lo and behold, *another* earthquake hit. Obviously this would further damage the structure, making it weaker, not stronger, right?

The take-home message is that the objective of your workout is to get this process started—to set this magic in motion. But remember, it is between workouts that your body rebuilds itself. It is between workouts that your muscles repair themselves, growing stronger and firmer each time. It is between workouts that you must fuel your body with the proper nutrients to feed your muscles. And it is between workouts that you must allow yourself time to rest and relax to ensure proper recovery.

bodyforlife.com   www.bodyforlife.com   www.bodyforlife.com   www.bodyforlife.com   www.bodyforlife.com   www.bodyforlife

Myth: Lifting a weight is what stimulates muscle growth.
Fact: Lifting *and* lowering a weight stimulates muscle growth.

In any free-weight exercise, there are two basic motions. One is called the concentric (lifting) phase; the other, the eccentric (lowering). During the concentric phase of an exercise, the muscle shortens or contracts. During the eccentric phase, just the opposite happens—the muscle lengthens.

A prime example is the bench press. When you lift the weight, pressing it from your chest to the lock-out position, that's the concentric or positive phase of the exercise; when you lower the weight from the lock-out position to the chest, that's the eccentric or negative portion of the exercise.

Enough evidence now exists to concretely state that lowering the weight is just as important as lifting it. It's true. It turns out that weight lowering causes much of the muscle-cell damage that stimulates an adaptation. You see, when you lengthen the muscle, which occurs during that eccentric portion of an exercise, you literally tear portions of the muscle fibers, signaling a stage of remodeling, or muscle growth. (You'll know when you've experienced this phenomenon because a day or two after your workout, your muscles will be sore. That's a sign that the "earth has moved.")

So, when you lift those barbells and dumbbells, keep in mind that you should not just haphazardly let gravity return it to its starting position. Always, and I repeat, *always* contract your muscles during the eccentric phase of an exercise—always let the weight down smoothly and slowly. If you don't, you're simply wasting your time.

The bottom line is, you must focus on lifting *and* lowering those weights.

Myth: A certain number of sets and reps gets the job done.
Fact: High-intensity effort produces the best results.

Let me say right here that everyone can benefit from even the most casual weight-training program. Any amount of resistance exercise, no matter how

bodyforlife.com   www.bodyforlife.com   www.bodyforlife.com   www.bodyforlife.com   www.bodyforlife.com   www.bodyforlife

small, can improve your overall health, help you burn calories, and even improve your mood. Regularly training with weights is a very enjoyable activity that can help build anyone's self-esteem.

I'll say it again—any exercise is better than no exercise.

But, if your goal is to make a significant transformation, you're going to have to focus on pushing yourself further than you may ever have pushed yourself before.

You are going to have to train with *heart and soul.*

I'm not just talking about working out "hard." Nor am I referring to how many hours a week you spend in the gym. I'm talking about finding something in yourself you don't know—or don't believe—is there. I'm talking about pushing yourself beyond limits you might think right now are unbendable.

Many people who work out with weights, who don't get results, overlook this fact. They simply don't train intensely enough to push their bodies to the point where their muscles will be forced to adapt and grow. Most people *think* they are pushing themselves enough. But they *aren't.*

Remember, perception is reality. Nowhere is this lesson more clearly understood, nowhere are "limits" more amazingly redefined, than with resistance training. And no lesson you learn or skill you develop in that weight room will be more powerfully applied to the rest of your life than this one: The limits you are living with right now, in every aspect of your existence, have been created by your mind. They are perceptions. And they are holding you back. You are capable of far more than you think you are.

The question is whether you are prepared to begin breaking through and discovering the far reaches of your true potential. That, again, is what this book—the techniques I've already laid out and the Program to which those tools will be applied—is all about, both with the body and beyond.

With resistance training and *life*, the simple, inescapable fact is that maximum intensity occurs *after* you have "perceived" failure. Those who can go beyond that—to a higher point—to push themselves to a place where they have not been before are the ones who will experience dramatic results, *fast.*

bodyforlife.com   www.bodyforlife.com   www.bodyforlife.com   www.bodyforlife.com   www.bodyforlife.com   www.bodyforlife

Myth: To lose fat, and improve your body, don't eat.
Fact: To build a lean, healthy body, you *have* to eat!

One of the most crucial errors people make when they try to lose fat and improve their health is severely restricting food intake. That doesn't work. It never works. If you try to "starve off" unwanted fat, you are playing a game you can't win. To get the best results, you need to work *with* your body, not *against* it.

You see, our bodies have been forged through tens of thousands of years of evolution. Our "genetic programming" gives our bodies the ability to control the production of enzymes, which, in turn, control every aspect of our metabolism. Due to this fact, your body will "fight back" when you severely reduce food intake—it decreases the rate at which it burns fat. (Your genetic coding has no idea there's a McDonald's, Burger King, or convenience store within walking distance. That coding assumes a food shortage or famine has just hit.)

Okay, so now you know one of your body's "survival mechanisms" is to lower your metabolic rate when you starve it. But that's not all that happens. You also begin to lose muscle tissue. You'll feel tired, weak, and irritable. Your immune system will suffer, too. And you'll develop nutrient deficiencies that will cause literally thousands of your body's natural metabolic processes to misfire. Within days, your body will sound the alarm: "emergency . . . emergency . . . eat, eat, eat." The next thing you know, you're bingeing on everything in sight: cookies, ice cream, chips, cereal, and more cookies.

People who force themselves to stick with a crash diet will lose body weight, but it's a very unfavorable type of weight loss. Typically, half of the pounds lost come from muscle tissue that is sacrificed. It's very important to remember muscle is your body's metabolic furnace. Muscle uses energy, even while you're sleeping. Fat pretty much just sits there.

To make matters worse, when you do go off the diet (which everyone who goes on a very low-calorie diet does at some point), you will gain back the fat you lost, and *more*. That's because you've turned your body into a less efficient

.bodyforlife.com   www.bodyforlife.com   www.bodyforlife.com   www.bodyforlife.com   www.bodyforlife.com   www.bodyforlife

fat-burning machine by losing muscle. (Now you can eat less and still gain fat—what a great plan!) When you try to lose fat again, you'll have to eat even *less* to drop weight. But eventually you'll give in and gain back even more fat. This frightening process is what is popularly described as "yo-yo dieting."

Perhaps you've tried to get lean by following a very low-calorie diet, and maybe you've experienced some of the adverse effects I described above. I sure have. And I can tell you, it's no fun. I felt out of control and unstable. I became weaker mentally and physically. Fortunately, I found a better way—the right way.

What I discovered is that it is possible to lose fat without losing muscle; in fact, you can lose fat, gain muscle, and improve your mental and physical strength at the same time. And you can do it in as little as 12 weeks. But, to make that breakthrough, you *must* let go of the myth that not eating is the key to fat loss. You *must* accept that you need plenty of good quality nutrition to build a better body.

Myth: Eating right means three "square meals" a day.
Fact: Eating *six* nutritious meals a day is the *right way*!

Okay, so now you know why starving yourself does not work and that eating isn't just "allowed," it's a must. The next myth that stands in the way is that three square meals a day are all you need.

I don't know exactly where that idea of three is best comes from, but it wasn't the way our ancestors ate. If you look at how humans evolved, you'll see our long-lost relatives were "frequent feeders," not bingers.

It's revealing to take a look at the animal kingdom and notice the relationship between creatures' eating patterns and their body "types." At one end of the spectrum are animals that load up on large amounts of food at one "meal," then go for days, weeks, or even months without eating at all. Bears are a prime example of this type of infrequent feeder. They're what I call *bingers*. They have huge body-fat storage compartments to stockpile the fuel they'll need to

bodyforlife.com   www.bodyforlife.com   www.bodyforlife.com   www.bodyforlife.com   www.bodyforlife.com   www.bodyforlife.

carry them from one feeding to the next. At the other end of the eating-pattern spectrum are the frequent feeders: animals that eat almost constantly but in far lesser amounts. Horses, buffalo, elk—I call these *grazers*. Relatively speaking, they have very low body fat and lots of lean muscle.

It seems pretty clear that we should graze, not binge, don't you think?

So, just how often should you eat? The answer is more often than you do now. To transform your body—to look better, feel better, and improve your health, you must develop the pattern of feeding your body frequently throughout the day—of grazing. You should not go more than a few hours (while you're awake) without eating. There are many reasons for this. One is that eating often helps keep your body's "food alarm" in check—it helps convince your body and mind there is not a famine around the corner. Also, studies show eating often helps accelerate the metabolism, so you burn more calories. And when you graze—when you eat six nutritious, smaller meals a day—the food is more efficiently absorbed and processed by your body than the "three squares" most Americans eat each day.

When you eat every few hours, you'll have more energy, less hunger pangs and cravings, and I'm certain you'll just flat out feel better—a lot better. On top of all that, you'll be creating a "metabolic environment" that supports healthy fat loss and muscle gains.

Myth: People who overeat lack willpower.
Fact: Overeating is a natural instinct.

Hard as it might be for some people to believe, human beings haven't always been able to summon all the food they can eat over the phone or from the driver's seat of a car. Long before there were phones or cars (long, as in tens of thousands of years ago), our ancestors did not have a consistently abundant supply of food. They were hunters/gatherers and, more recently, farmers, who sometimes had plenty to eat but regularly endured periods of time when there was little or nothing to eat. This selective pressure forced their bodies to

,bodyforlife.com   www.bodyforlife.com   www.bodyforlife.com   www.bodyforlife.com   www.bodyforlife.com   www.bodyforlife

develop an almost unlimited ability to store excess energy in the form of body fat and very adaptive metabolisms to cope with periods of different diets.

And that has created a problem. Our bodies are still governed by this "survival mechanism," which is now backfiring in a world where eating has become easy. Quite simply—and tragically—people in this country have become victims of the industrialized food revolution. Everywhere you go, there's food, food, food. You can get a pizza and cheeseburger in just about every airport, train station, sports arena, hotel, street corner . . . just about anywhere. Everywhere you can possibly go, food will be there—waiting, begging, tempting you, and luring you in.

Letting our hunter/gatherer instinct—that primitive genetic coding—control our eating patterns has put us in a real sticky situation. I call modern America the nation of the *overfed and undernourished*. We are overfed on empty calories. Overfed on unhealthy saturated fat. Overfed on carbohydrates. Underfed on protein. Underfed on vitamins and minerals. Underfed on nutrients that help sustain life. And overfed on junk that takes life away.

The bottom line is, our natural instincts, combined with a food distribution system that's gone mad, are partly to blame for this bulging crisis.

However, just because it's "natural" to overeat doesn't mean it's unavoidable. Knowing the enemy is an important component of winning this battle.

Myth: High-carbohydrate, low-fat diets work best.
Fact: People are becoming fat from a "carb overdose."

In recent years, there have been so many different diets—so many different ways of "eating right"—that it's mind-boggling. However, the one which seems to have "stuck," the one that seems to be recommended and followed more often than any other, is a high-carbohydrate, low-fat, low-protein nutrition plan. This type of diet is recommended by many nutritionists and even some doctors.

bodyforlife.com   www.bodyforlife.com   www.bodyforlife.com   www.bodyforlife.com   www.bodyforlife.com   www.bodyforlife

One reason these high-carb, low-fat diets are so popular is because back in 1988, the U.S. Surgeon General recommended we all restrict our consumption of dietary fat, and in response, the multibillion-dollar food industry began coming out with fat-free everything—ice cream, cookies, crackers, you name it. In place of fat, more and more carbs were added. And the myth that "fat free" means "all you can eat" spread like wildfire. But yet, over the past 10 years, we've continued to see a dramatic rise in the incidence of obesity.

The fact is, lowering your dietary fat intake and increasing carbohydrate consumption is not the best way to get lean and healthy. It's not the best way to ward off many of the health-related problems associated with not eating right either.

I've worked with a lot of people over the years who were consuming a low-fat, high-carb diet and exercising, but they were getting even *fatter!* When I informed them that their diets were all wrong, they argued vehemently that their way was the best way. (This myth is a stubborn one.)

Folks, I don't know everything about everything, but I'm certain of what I'm certain of, and I'm certain that following a high-carbohydrate diet is not going to help you transform your physique, improve your health, and help you build a stronger, healthier, more energetic body.

Remember those long-lost ancestors of ours I keep telling you about? The ones who were hunters/gatherers? Well, they ate a very protein-rich diet. They didn't eat cookies and crackers and candy. And, according to anthropologists, they were strong, had well-formed bones, strong teeth, and they were rarely overly fat.

However, about 8,000 years ago, the Egyptians learned to farm and shifted over to consuming more carbohydrates, primarily in the form of grains. And, according to experts, the health of these ancient folks began to decline. But why? According to today's "high carbs is best" myth, the Egyptians should have been healthier and more fit. However, that's not the way it worked out. They actually became an obese society with widespread heart disease, stunted growth, and malnutrition.

.bodyforlife.com   www.bodyforlife.com   www.bodyforlife.com   www.bodyforlife.com   www.bodyforlife.com   www.bodyforlife

The fact is, our bodies work much better with a balance of carbohydrates and protein. You see, not only is protein essential for building healthy muscles and maintaining a strong immune system but it helps stabilize insulin levels as well. Insulin is what I call a "nutrient-transport hormone." It shuttles amino acids and glucose (blood sugar), among other things, into cells. But, when you eat too many carbs over a long period of time, your body becomes "insulin resistant," and you can develop adult-onset diabetes, which can lead to obesity, heart disease, and a whole lot of other health problems, including unstable energy levels and fatigue. Eating a high-carb diet can also stimulate the appetite and cause unfavorable and unpredictable mood swings (especially in the midafternoon). Moreover, whenever insulin levels are elevated, your body will not burn fat.

On the other hand, protein provides stable energy levels through its effect on insulin and blood sugar. Eating protein also helps control your appetite. And research has found that the thermic effect (the increase in energy required for digestion, absorption, and disposal of ingested food) of a protein-rich meal is much greater than a high-carbohydrate meal.

I could go on and on about this topic, but the bottom line is, high-carbo-hydrate diets work against the body, not with it. The solution is to balance carbohydrate and protein intake.

Myth: Eating right means avoiding bad foods.
Fact: You must avoid bad foods and consume good foods.

Many people know that eating too much of certain foods is unhealthy. Yet what remains "undiscovered" by so many is that you not only need to avoid the bad stuff, you need to eat the good stuff. You see, the good stuff can help you as much or more than the bad stuff can hurt you.

It was Hippocrates, the founding father of modern medicine, who, a couple thousand years ago, said, "Let food be your medicine, and let medicine be your food." What Hippocrates understood, and what's crucial for each of

bodyforlife.com   www.bodyforlife.com   www.bodyforlife.com   www.bodyforlife.com   www.bodyforlife.com   www.bodyforlife.

us to realize as we seriously turn our attention to what we eat, is that we can either overdose on the wrong kinds of food or we can consume a healthy "prescription" of foods that contain the nutrients our bodies need. The fact, which is being overlooked by so many, is that there are nutrients in certain foods that, when consumed regularly and in the proper amounts, allow the body to be its own best "pharmacy"—to protect and heal itself.

So remember this: Virtually all foods have "druglike" effects—they can improve your health or destroy it. For example, if you feed your body consistently with an abundant supply of nutrients that act as antioxidants, you can significantly lower your risk of getting certain types of cancer. On the other hand, if you overdose on foods rich in saturated fat, you can suffer deadly side effects such as heart disease. Thus, we should focus not just on avoiding bad foods but we must continually nourish our bodies with good foods like the ones I'll tell you about later in this book.

Myth: You have to count every calorie you eat.
Fact: You should count "portions," not calories.

All right, by now you know that eating frequently is important, and you've also been made aware of the significance of consuming a balance of protein and carbohydrates. By this point, if you're like most folks I work with, you're wondering when it's going to get complicated—when I'm going to mandate that you count every calorie you eat or perhaps even require that you weigh your food on a little scale and all that jazz.

Well, if that's what you're waiting for, keep waiting because it ain't gonna happen. You see, I've learned that most people in the real world don't count calories. They just won't do it.

The solution? We count "portions" instead.

"What's a portion?" you ask.

Well, a portion is an amount of food roughly equal to the size of your clenched fist or the palm of your hand. For example, if a baked potato is about

bodyforlife.com   www.bodyforlife.com   www.bodyforlife.com   www.bodyforlife.com   **www.bodyforlife.com**   www.bodyforlife

the size of your clenched fist, that's a portion for you. If a chicken breast is about the size of the palm of your hand, that's your portion of chicken.

It's really quite simple to follow the portion rule once you get the hang of it. As long as the foods you select are low in fat (like baked potatoes, steamed brown rice, broiled salmon, grilled chicken breasts, and other healthy foods you'll learn about later in this book), you can't go wrong.

Myth: If you "eat right," you don't need to take supplements.
Fact: Studies show many of us do need to take supplements.

Despite what some "old-school" dietitians and other "experts" might tell you, there really is a very sound, scientific basis for supplementation. In fact, even the National Institutes of Health (NIH) has recognized the role of nutritional supplements in physically active people's nutrition plans.

Consider this: Even if you had a full-time personal chef in your kitchen, or if you were able to spend all day, every day doing nothing but shopping for and preparing the "best" regular-food meals, you still couldn't be certain you were getting all the nutrients your body needs.

You see, the amount of nutrients such as the vitamin C found in two seemingly identical oranges at your local grocery store can vary enormously. How long ago was the fruit picked? What type of soil was it grown in? (Much of the soil in the United States is deficient in essential nutrients.) What part of the country did it come from?

It's impossible to predict the nutrient value of various whole foods. And even if you did know exactly what everything contained, it's impractical (if not impossible) for most people to get all the nutrients their bodies require to function optimally from regular food without consuming far more calories than they need. That's why I've used vitamin and mineral supplements, as well as nutrition shakes, virtually every day for the last 10 years. I also recommend supplements to the athletes, actors, doctors, lawyers, moms, and dads—*all* the people I work with.

bodyforlife.com　www.bodyforlife.com　www.bodyforlife.com　www.bodyforlife.com　www.bodyforlife.com　www.bodyforlife.

Myth: You need to drink water only when you are thirsty.
Fact: Your body needs more water than it's telling you.

Healthy muscle is comprised of more than 70 percent water. And water is an essential transport mechanism for a vast array of nutrients like vitamins and minerals and even carbohydrates. It serves an important role in all cellular activity. If your water intake is low, your ability to transport nutrients becomes compromised, and you'll lose strength and feel sluggish because of the buildup of ammonia, urea, uric acid, and other junk you don't want hanging around in your body.

Also, if you happen to be someone who struggles with water retention, one of the best ways to get rid of that is to drink more water, not less. Water retention is just another aspect of your body's survival mechanism.

Drinking water can also help you control your appetite. If you find that the portions of food you're eating don't quite satisfy you, try drinking a cup of water before you even take your first bite of food. Then drink another cup of water with your meal. You'll find this helps alleviate that feeling of not having eaten enough.

I can't overemphasize how important water is to your body's health and proper functioning. You need it constantly. I don't care if it's bottled or tap water. Drink it with meals and between them. Drink it often, and drink a lot.

Myth: You have to eat "perfectly" all the time.
Fact: There's no such thing as eating "perfectly."

Don't be too hard on yourself if you end up eating too much or not often enough one day. If you do, just put it behind you and get back on schedule. Don't beat yourself up, and don't *ever* give up on yourself.

It's so disappointing for me to see people who are making excellent progress—who are well on their way to a successful transformation—then they eat something they shouldn't, or they miss a workout, and they just quit.

bodyforlife.com   www.bodyforlife.com   www.bodyforlife.com   www.bodyforlife.com   www.bodyforlife.com   www.bodyforlife

Please don't do this!

Keep in mind that I have yet to meet a real-life transformation champion, including all those you'll read about in this book, who didn't "mess up" from time to time. They succeeded because they persevered, *not* because they were perfect.

So if you stumble once in a while, just put it behind you and resolve to do better from that point forward. The mere fact that you have decided to improve yourself is something to be proud of. Focus on that.

And, when those cravings hit, *which they will*, remember that *nothing tastes as good as being in the greatest shape of your life feels*. Also remember it's just food. *You control it*. It doesn't control you.

Accept the fact that no one is perfect, yet we *all* have the potential to improve—we all have the power to change.

With that in mind, let's now move onward *and upward*.

bodyforlife.com   www.bodyforlife.com   www.bodyforlife.com   www.bodyforlife.com   www.bodyforlife.com   www.bodyforlife

Overview of Separating Myth from Fact

Myth: Aerobics is better for shaping up than weight training.
Fact: To transform your physique, you *must* train with weights.

Myth: If you exercise, it doesn't matter what you eat.
Fact: If you exercise, it matters *even more* what you eat.

Myth: If women lift weights, they'll get "bulky."
Fact: Resistance exercise helps women create lean, toned bodies.

Myth: Weight training is only for young athletes.
Fact: People of all ages should be weight training.

Myth: Muscles grow while you're working out.
Fact: Muscles grow while you're resting and recuperating.

Myth: A certain number of sets and reps gets the job done.
Fact: High-intensity effort produces the best results.

Myth: Eating right means three "square meals" a day.
Fact: Eating *six* nutritious meals a day is the *right way*!

Myth: People who overeat lack willpower.
Fact: Overeating is a natural instinct.

Myth: High-carbohydrate, low-fat diets work best.
Fact: People are becoming fat from a "carb overdose."

Myth: You have to count every calorie you eat.
Fact: You should count "portions," not calories.

Myth: If you "eat right," you don't need to take supplements.
Fact: Studies show many of us do need to take supplements.

Myth: You need to drink water only when you are thirsty.
Fact: Your body needs more water than it's telling you.

Myth: You have to eat "perfectly" all the time.
Fact: There's no such thing as eating "perfectly."

w.bodyforlife.com   www.bodyforlife.com   www.bodyforlife.com   www.bodyforlife.com   **www.bodyforlife.com**   www.bodyforli

The Training-*for*-LIFE Experience™

─────────── Part IV ───────────

*When you overcome resistance, you create
the power to continually reach higher.*

Over the last decade, I've had the opportunity to work with and learn from some of the world's best athletic trainers and strength coaches, including Mike Woicik, who trained the Dallas Cowboys during their world-champion seasons in 1993 and 1994; Tim Grover, Sports Enhancement Specialist for athletes such as Michael Jordan; and many others. I've also been fortunate to work with and learn from some of the world's leading doctors, physiologists, and scientists, including Eric Hultman, Ph.D., of the world-renown Karolinska Institute in Sweden.

And, as I've previously explained, I've learned *so* much from the thousands of real-life champions who have shared their successes and setbacks with me. I've also used my own body as a testing ground—trying all these different exercise techniques and carefully monitoring and measuring the results, not just on my muscle size and strength and body-fat levels but also on how each routine affected the way I *feel*—my ability to focus at work, my energy levels, and my clarity.

I've taken everything I've learned, everything I've felt, and everything I know and assimilated it, synthesized it, and created a unique, powerful transformation method, which I call the Training-*for*-LIFE Experience.

55

It's not merely an exercise routine. It is, as its name indicates, an experience. By that, I mean you don't *just* do it. You live *it*.

Everything about the Training-*for*-LIFE Experience is based on tried and true principles which have been precisely formulated to help stimulate increases in muscle and strength, as well as burn body fat. In addition, every time you have this experience, you'll be training yourself to set and achieve goals, practice positive patterns of action, increase focus, overcome resistance, and become a stronger person in every way imaginable.

The Training-*for*-LIFE Experience is based on universal principles which have already produced breakthroughs for tens of thousands of people. It *will* benefit virtually any healthy adult, regardless of his or her level of fitness. I'm not saying it's the only approach that works, but I guarantee when you follow it to the letter, you *will* get results. That's because anatomically and physiologically, every human being is essentially the same, and although certain genetic factors do vary, that does not mean each and every person needs his or her own custom-made exercise program. Quite literally, the same Program that works for me also works for my mom, my co-workers, my friends—*everyone*.

The Training-*for*-LIFE Experience is not only effective but efficient—it requires *only* two percent of the time you have available to you every week. You do *not* have to turn your life upside down to fit this into your daily routine. In fact, when you begin following this Program, you'll quickly find it doesn't take time, it *creates* time—it is so precise and so focused that it will enhance your energy and clarity, enabling you to fit more into your personal and professional life. Performing this unique type of exercise regularly can even extend the active, enjoyable, rewarding years of your life. In that way, it can not only help you create a few extra hours a week, it can literally add years—active, fun, *fulfilling* years—to your time in this world.

The Training-*for*-LIFE Experience may very well be the most practical and result-producing exercise Program there is. In fact, I believe this breakthrough will, by the last day of 2001, help one million people transform their bodies and lives.

Let's take a look at the techniques that make it so effective.

odyforlife.com   www.bodyforlife.com   www.bodyforlife.com   www.bodyforlife.com   www.bodyforlife.com   www.bodyforlife.c

Plan-to-Actual Analysis

One of the keys to our success will be our meticulous planning. Before we begin each training session, we'll know what exercises we're going to perform, how many sets, the number of reps, and how much weight we're going to use. We'll even plan precisely how long, from beginning to end, we will be training. Therefore, we'll move swiftly from one exercise to the next with a clear sense of purpose.

We *never* just go "work out" without having planned it beforehand. This is a mistake so many people make. You'll see them walking around in the gym, scratching their heads, obviously trying to figure out what they should do next. (Sadly, this is probably the way they live their lives as well.) Often, they'll take a look at what someone else is doing and copy that. Unfortunately, what they don't know is that the other people, whose actions they're imitating, don't know what they're doing either! It's the blind leading (or misleading) the blind. Folks, this is the antithesis of the Training-*for*-LIFE approach: What these people are doing is completely arbitrary—it is trial and error, and, in actuality, it is a waste of time.

To help guide you step by step, day by day, through every aspect of the spectacular journey you're about to begin, I have included your first week's "Daily Progress Reports" (see pages 175–187). This way, you can plan, record, and analyze your training and measure your progress. Don't use your Progress Reports just to keep track of where you've been—use them to plan where you're going.

Through your records, you can clearly see the path you're on. If you're not transforming as rapidly as you would like, you can go back and troubleshoot, with precision. Are you making it to each exercise session? Are you hitting the appropriate intensity levels? Are you doing too much or not enough? These are the types of questions you'll be able to ask and answer when you keep a detailed journal.

And, when you do make rapid progress, you'll have a record of it so you can repeat the activities that are working. I've learned from past experience

.bodyforlife.com   www.bodyforlife.com   www.bodyforlife.com   www.bodyforlife.com   www.bodyforlife.com   www.bodyforlife

that the only thing worse than working hard and not getting anywhere is getting results and not knowing how you got them. You see, if you go from point A to point B and you don't know how you got there, you're still lost.

It takes less than 10 minutes a day to keep your records up to date. It's unquestionably one of the most important exercises you can do to ensure your success.

The High-Point Technique™

You don't need any fancy equipment to perform The Training-*for*-LIFE Experience exercises I explain in the Exercise Guide on page 135. As you'll discover, these exercises are very basic. You can do most of them with a simple set of barbells and dumbbells in a home gym or virtually any fitness center.

You see, it's not so much *what* exercises we do but rather *how* we do them that matters most. We *must* perform these exercises *intensely* to produce rapid results. Which brings us to what I call the "High-Point Technique." It's based on something I discovered while working in the magazine business for the last seven years.

Let me explain . . . I've worked with a lot of photographers and helped direct many photo shoots over the years. Sometimes you shoot for 11 hours and don't end up with any cover-worthy photos. It can be quite frustrating. You work hard all day but end up with nothing. That's the way it goes with most of the photographers I've worked with.

Fortunately, there are a few exceptions—some photographers take an entirely different approach. They begin with a quick, calculated setup. Then, they find their position, take a "warm-up" photo or two, and proceed to capture the "moment" on film. That's it. Photo shoot over.

And the result? Well, if you've seen the photos on covers of magazines like *Sports Illustrated, People, Time,* or even my magazine, you can see that the results are impressive. Sometimes breathtaking.

bodyforlife.com   www.bodyforlife.com   www.bodyforlife.com   www.bodyforlife.com   www.bodyforlife.com   www.bodyforlife.

How can such extraordinary results be created in so little time? Why are most photographers, who work for hours . . . even days . . . unable to produce photos of comparable quality?

I believe what makes these photographers so effective is that they know how to capture the "moment that matters." A moment called the "high point."

What's this have to do with getting a good workout? A lot, actually.

You see, when you get right down to it, not only is a successful photo shoot contingent on hitting a high point, so is a great workout, so is a productive day at work, and . . . so is a fulfilling life.

Those moments when everything comes together and you reach higher than you've ever reached—when you do something you've never done—when you produce major results—it's those moments that define who and where you are.

Do you have a scrapbook with photos of yourself and your family in it? If so, what exactly do you have in there? Do you have pictures of yourself getting dressed in the morning? A snapshot of you tying your shoe? Driving to work? Sitting at your desk shuffling through papers? Grocery shopping? Probably not.

My guess is that your scrapbook is filled with pictures that reflect special moments. Standing on top of a mountain peak. Your wedding day. Your child's first step. Winning an award. A celebration. A vivid smile on a loved one's face that makes you smile and gives you energy just thinking about it. These moments are all "high points," right?

Think about it: Superman's "super moments" are his high points. The rest—his life as Clark Kent—is pretty forgettable.

For athletes like Joe Montana, Michael Jordan, John Elway, and Mark McGwire, the moments that define their greatness are their high points.

I'm sure you've got the picture by now. It's really not a hard concept to grasp, once someone makes you aware of it. Unfortunately, most people aren't consciously aware of the power of high points, so it's impossible for them to create "moments that matter." The few high points most people experience occur randomly—by accident. And that's not good. For our exercise sessions to create major results fast, we must learn to recognize high points and create them.

.bodyforlife.com   www.bodyforlife.com   www.bodyforlife.com   www.bodyforlife.com   www.bodyforlife.com   www.bodyforlife

It's About *Quality*, Not Quantity

When you develop the skill to intentionally create high points, you can not only experience more energy and greater success in life, you can also produce major results in minimal time, in any area. So, that's the way I work. It's also the way I work out.

However, many "fitness experts" recommend that as soon as you can exercise for 30 minutes "comfortably," you should increase to 40 minutes. Then 60. Then 90. "More is better," they proclaim.

My question to them is, "*Why?*"

What's the objective, to eventually work out all day? Gee, that sounds swell, but I was kind of hoping I could get in shape *and* have a life.

Think about it, if more were better, for those great photographers to improve, a photo session that took an hour when they were "beginners" would now take them a week.

The fact of the matter is, as you become more experienced—as your level of expertise in whatever it is you're doing, including exercise, advances—the objective is to continually reach higher and become even more efficient.

You see, once you learn that skill—once you develop the ability to create higher and higher high points—you will not only experience continual progress, you'll be downright unstoppable. That's what keeps you growing. It's what keeps you excited. It's what keeps you feeling alive. These moments create momentum, and once you get this process started, you'll start making breakthroughs you never imagined.

And that's why I do not recommend you work out for hours and hours on end. We set up, we prime our minds and bodies, and then we focus on creating a high point.

Sound a bit mystical? Well, let's look at it from a scientific standpoint for a moment. During our workouts, we're trying to stimulate an adaptation response. Well, guess what? Studies show that the stimulation required to trigger muscle growth happens fast or not at all. Hence, the maxim, "You can work out hard or long." It's one or the other.

bodyforlife.com   www.bodyforlife.com   www.bodyforlife.com   www.bodyforlife.com   www.bodyforlife.com   www.bodyforlife.

Also, keep in mind the body has a limited ability to recover from physical activity; therefore, if you continue to engage in moderate- or low-intensity exercise, after you hit the high point, you will be short-circuiting your progress because you'll be overextending your body's recuperative ability. It's imperative to realize that a high point is just that—it's a point. It's not a plateau. It's not a "level place" you get to. You can't maintain a high point. You can be there only for an instant.

Therefore, for each workout, I'm going to ask you to perform only a few bursts of maximally intense exercise. These sets will be challenging. Each week I will ask you to raise the bar another notch—to push yourself to a higher point. I'm not asking for your "best effort." I want more than that. I believe your perception of what your best effort is may be a self-imposed limitation. I believe you are capable of much more than you realize, and now is the time to shatter those false barriers and discover your true potential.

Your High Point Is *Your* High Point

With the Training-*for*-LIFE Experience, we use a tool called the "Intensity Index" to help us create high points. This "meter" is used to measure the level of focused energy we are putting forth. The Index, shown on the following page, starts at level 1 and goes to level 10.

On the low end—at level 1—you've got the intensity of sitting on the couch watching TV. Level 2 would be standing; level 3 might be walking; level 4 might be carrying a couple bags of groceries in from the car; level 5 might be carrying those groceries up a flight of stairs; and so on, up to level 10, which is an all-out, 100 percent focused effort.

The proper use of the Intensity Index makes the Training-*for*-LIFE Experience, by design, self-regulating. And that's why virtually any healthy adult, regardless of prior exercise experience, can begin this Program. For example, if you're a beginner and you can bench press 30 pounds for 12 reps, that's your high-intensity effort. Now, someone who's been training for several

.bodyforlife.com   www.bodyforlife.com   www.bodyforlife.com   www.bodyforlife.com   www.bodyforlife.com   www.bodyforlife

The Intensity Index™

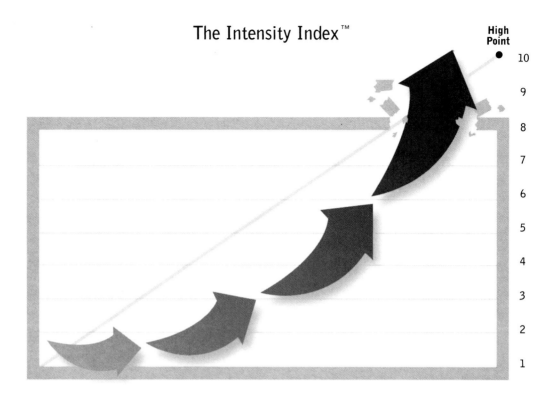

years might reach a high-intensity effort by bench pressing 185 pounds for 12 reps. The point is, your high point is *yours*. It is unique to you. As you adapt and evolve, so does this Program; in fact, you can never outgrow it.

It's very important you become aware of what your high points are. A true high point on this workout, a true level 10 experience, is one where you can honestly tell yourself you gave it every single last ounce of energy you had—that you tapped into your inner strength. What you'll discover is a true high point comes from your mind, not your muscles.

After you finish your highest intensity set (for that muscle group) and before you write down whether you had a level 8, level 9, or a level 10 experience, you need to answer this question: Could you have done one more rep if I were standing right there, encouraging you to reach even higher—to push yourself further?

62   Body-*for*-LIFE

If your honest answer is, "No way!" then congratulations! You scored a 10!

However, if your answer is something along the lines of, "Maybe I could have done another one," then you're probably looking at a 9. Which is a solid effort. Celebrate the progress you made, and plan to try even harder next time.

You won't reach a high point every time. That would be like John Elway expecting to throw a touchdown pass every time he touched the ball. You see, a high point is kind of like a touchdown pass—it's a challenge, which is why it's a worthwhile goal. Very few of the high points you hit in life are going to be easy.

With the Training-*for*-LIFE Experience, I'll indicate precisely when you should reach for your high points, and I'll ask you to rate your level of intensity. What we'll be doing is creating a wave-like pattern of intensity—always starting with a moderate level and rising toward a high point. The charts which follow show the desired Intensity Pattern for the upper and lower body training routines, which I'll walk you through later in this section.

The Upper Body Training Experience™

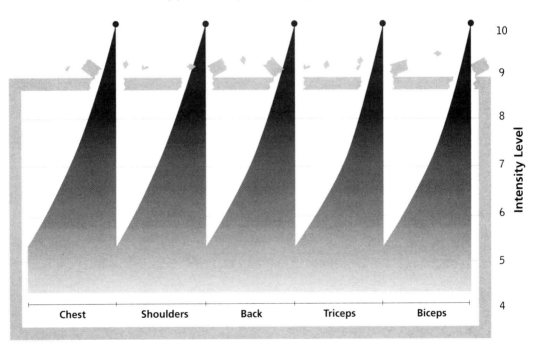

bodyforlife.com   www.bodyforlife.com   www.bodyforlife.com   www.bodyforlife.com   www.bodyforlife.com   www.bodyforlife

The Lower Body Training Experience™

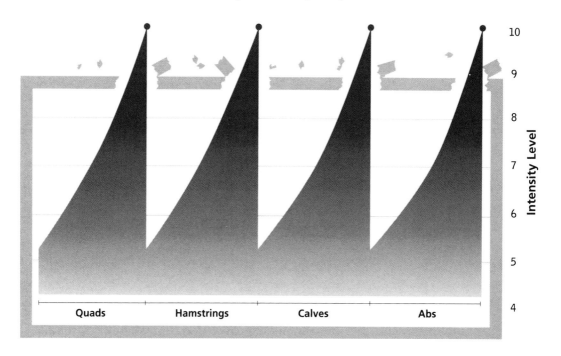

——— The 20-Minute Aerobics Solution™ ———

If you're like most people, you've probably done some, or maybe a lot of, aerobic exercise but haven't noticed too much of a difference. And the prospect of doing more isn't very appealing.

After all, if those long, boring, unfocused exercise routines—the type that so many millions of people conduct, week in and week out—worked, why do so darn many overweight women and men who take part in all those aerobic classes, month after month, look exactly the same now as they did a year ago?

Wouldn't it be great if there were an aerobics alternative—something much more efficient? Something that produced maximum results in minimum time?

Well, guess what? There is.

I call it the 20-Minute Aerobics Solution.

bodyforlife.com   www.bodyforlife.com   www.bodyforlife.com   www.bodyforlife.com   www.bodyforlife.com   www.bodyforlife.

It's a unique workout which incorporates the High-Point Technique and the Intensity Index, thus transforming ordinary aerobics into an extraordinary event that, like our weight-training routine, is both self-regulating and evolutionary. That means no matter what your present condition, you're ready for the 20-Minute Aerobics Solution. And you can never outgrow it.

Despite what so many millions of people have been told, low-intensity, long-duration aerobic exercise is not the best method for ridding the body of excess fat. You probably knew deep down, anyhow, that busting your behind burned off more fat than exercise that allowed you to take it easy, didn't you? Well, scientific studies and thousands of real-life examples now show your instincts were right.

You see, research indicates that not only does high-intensity training burn fat more effectively than low-intensity exercise—up to 50 percent more efficiently—it also speeds up your metabolism and keeps it revved up for some time after your workout. So forget about the "calories burned" readout on the stairstepper or stationary bike; on this Program, the majority of calories will be used up the hour after our workouts, provided we don't eat for one hour after our exercise sessions.

To further enhance the fat-burning effects of these workouts, do them in the morning, in a fasted state (before eating). Scientific studies indicate that fat is burned much faster—up to 300 percent faster—when you exercise in the morning as opposed to doing the same exercise in the afternoon. (By the way, if your primary goal is to lose body fat, consider doing your weight-training workouts in the morning on an empty stomach, too.)

This Program involves performing only 20 minutes of aerobic exercise three times per week—no more, no less. Your challenge is to make each of those workouts the most effective fat-burning, health-enhancing 20 minutes you possibly can. And to do that, you simply use the Intensity Index and follow the numbers on the chart on page 62.

Let me show you how simple this is: What we do is select an exercise like walking, jogging, riding a stationary bike, using a treadmill, etc. You can vary

bodyforlife.com   www.bodyforlife.com   www.bodyforlife.com   www.bodyforlife.com   **www.bodyforlife.com**   www.bodyforlife

your aerobic exercise every session if you want. For example, I often do my aerobic exercise at home on a stationary bike. Other times I walk or jog outside. And sometimes I use a treadmill. Just as long as it's the type of aerobic exercise that allows you to increase the intensity in intervals, it will work just fine.

We start with a two-minute set-up phase where we perform the activity at about a level 5 intensity. If you haven't been exercising regularly, you could reach level 5 on the Intensity Index by just walking. However, if you've been doing a lot of exercise, level 5 might be a pretty brisk jog. The important thing to remember is that your level 5 is *your* level 5, and my level 5 is *my* level 5.

Now, after two minutes at a level 5 effort, we're going to take it up a notch. When we reach a level 6 effort, we keep it there for one minute; then we increase the intensity of our effort, up to level 7 for one minute before taking it up another notch, to level 8, where we maintain for another minute; then we take it up to level 9. We maintain that high-intensity effort for one minute, and then take it all the way down to a level 6 again—a relatively moderate effort.

We repeat that pattern three times, but on the last cycle (between the eighteenth and the nineteenth minutes of this 20-minute workout), we don't stop at level 9—we try to reach a high point—we go for a 10! Then we bring it back to level 5 for a minute, and we're done.

The chart on the following page shows what the Intensity Pattern of the 20-Minute Aerobics Solution I just described looks like.

By the way, a "high-intensity effort" does not mean an all-out sprint. If you haven't tried to run all-out since you were a kid, you're in for a shock. Don't take off like you're fleeing from a burning building, or *you'll* burn out well before the twentieth minute.

For some, an intense effort may mean just walking up a hill. If that's the case, don't be at all discouraged. This Program is about improving—moving forward in a positive way, and that's something we all have the capability of doing, if we choose to do it.

Now remember, you won't have a level 10 experience every workout. But you must try to achieve a higher and higher level of performance, or you

.bodyforlife.com   www.bodyforlife.com   www.bodyforlife.com   www.bodyforlife.com   www.bodyforlife.com   www.bodyforlife

The 20-Minute Aerobics Solution™

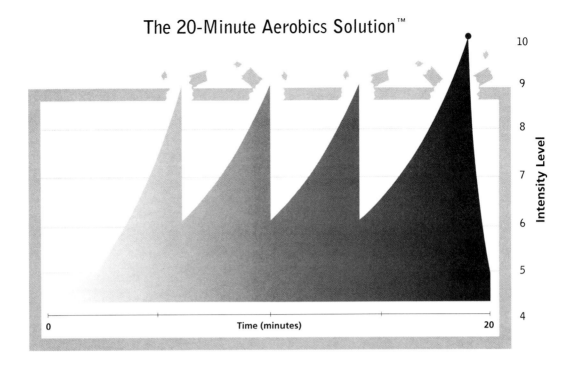

never will—you'll get stuck in the comfort zone, and your body will not be forced to adapt; therefore, even though you may be exercising regularly, you won't get results.

That's what happens to so many well-intentioned people who follow standard exercise routines—routines that are self-limiting by design. By that I mean they do *not* provide you with a plan or path that allows you to constantly improve. What many exercise routines do is actually "train you" to stay at a certain level. These programs don't evolve. They're static; they're stuck. (It's no wonder the people who follow those old-fashioned routines are stuck, too!)

Anyway, when you apply the Intensity Index properly to both your resistance training and aerobic workouts, you'll never hit the ceiling. You'll always move up to higher and higher high points. And that means you'll continually be stimulating your muscles while losing fat. You'll become more metabolically efficient. Your body will burn fat at a significantly elevated rate, even while you're sitting at your desk or driving your car or reading a book . . . even while you're sleeping.

.bodyforlife.com   www.bodyforlife.com   www.bodyforlife.com   www.bodyforlife.com   **www.bodyforlife.com**   www.bodyforlife

Sharing the Experience

So now we understand the importance of planning and keeping records. We've discovered a powerful, new growth strategy in the High-Point Technique. We've also seen how using the Intensity Index will help us make continual progress. However, we're not quite done yet. In order to help you understand how to put it all together, I'm going to share with you how I use the Training-*for*-LIFE tools and techniques to build my body for life.

Ready? Then let's do it.

I start by planning the coming day's workout the night before—in this case, Sunday night. I can tell by looking at my schedule that Monday is going to be a wild ride. I've got meetings, dozens of memos to write, two articles I need to finish for my next magazine, and I know enough to expect the unexpected. Mondays are almost always the most challenging, so I'm going to plan to do my upper body weight-training workout in the morning—that way I'll be sure to get it done, and I won't have to think about it all day.

So anyway, I plan my workout. I use the same Training-*for*-LIFE Daily Progress Report forms I'm making available to you. I've enclosed a page from my journal on page 73.

Notice that all I have to plan are the exercises I'm going to do and the weight I plan to use. The pattern of repetitions, the time I rest between sets, and the Intensity Pattern are always the same.

It takes me only about five minutes to plan my workout. I highly recommend you do the same thing I do—take just a few minutes the night before and think about when would be the best time for you to work out that next day. Then, plan which exercises you're going to do and what weight you're going to use.

Now, if you and I were doing this workout together and you weren't exactly sure which weight you should use for an exercise—the dumbbell bench press for example—what I'd do is hand you a pair of 10-pound dumbbells and let you do your first set with those. If it were really easy (like a level 3 intensity), you would not put the weights down and pick up a heavier set and

bodyforlife.com   www.bodyforlife.com   www.bodyforlife.com   www.bodyforlife.com   www.bodyforlife.com   www.bodyforlife.c

do another set of 12. You would write down, on your Daily Progress Report, under the "Actual" column, what weight you used and what intensity level it required. The next time you train the muscles of the upper body, you would be able to look back to this workout and see you need to use more weight. I'd suggest trying 20-pound dumbbells the next time. If that's still not a level 5 intensity—a moderate effort—the next time you would try 30-pound dumbbells. And, of course, if you overshoot the mark—if you select a weight that is too heavy, you can come back down five pounds. It's a fine-tuning process, but you'll get the hang of it, quickly.

My Inner-Strength Challenge

Fast-forward to Monday morning: I wake up at about 6:00 A.M. I throw on some shorts, a comfortable cotton T-shirt, and tennis shoes and drink two cups of water. I always drink water as soon as I get up in the morning because I haven't had any for at least six to eight hours, and my body needs it—water is so important to our health.

Today I'm going to work out at my house. I have an extra bedroom where I have a set of dumbbells, a workout bench, and a barbell. I also consider a stopwatch an important piece of equipment for my workouts. You should get one.

I start my chest workout with the dumbbell bench press by taking a 40-pound dumbbell in each hand. I lie back on the bench and press the weights up with a cadence of "Body-*for*-LIFE." I hold the dumbbells in the top position for a count of one, and then I lower them, slowly, as I say, "I am building my Body-*for*-LIFE." I pause just for a count of one at the bottom part of the exercise, and then I press the weights back up.

Forty-pound dumbbells, for me, are pretty light, but remember, I'm shooting for only a level 5 intensity rating. That means it's not even close to an all-out effort. I'm getting the blood flowing, getting my muscles warmed up, and clearing the fog from my mind. Remember, I just got out of bed a few minutes ago.

.bodyforlife.com   www.bodyforlife.com   www.bodyforlife.com   www.bodyforlife.com   www.bodyforlife.com   www.bodyforlife

After my set, I hit a stopwatch. I wait one minute, then pick up a couple of 50-pound dumbbells and perform 10 reps. It's a little more intense, but I could have done quite a few more reps. I wait one minute, then grab a set of 60-pound dumbbells, perform eight reps, which, for me, requires a level 7 effort. After waiting for another minute, I go up to 70-pound dumbbells for six reps.

By now, I've broken a sweat, and I've also fired up something called the neuromuscular junction, which is the point where our muscles receive a signal from our brains to flex. These signals are carried by neurotransmitters and flow through your nervous system like electricity flows through wires. It takes a few sets to get this neuromuscular junction primed. But once it's amped up and delivering full voltage, we will be stronger on the fifth set of an exercise in this workout—you'll be able to lift a weight 12 times that you might have been able to lift only eight times earlier in the workout. This system, however, is primed only for a brief period—there's a pretty small window of opportunity. That's why I designed the set and rep pattern the way I did. (See my example Daily Progress Report on page 73.) And that's why we must move swiftly, no time for idle chitchat with this Program.

Throughout the workout, I keep an eye on the clock to make sure I'm on schedule. My goal is to finish within 46 minutes. Having a deadline instills a sense of urgency and keeps me focused on my mission.

By this point, my mind and muscles are ready for my high-intensity effort. I pick up those 60-pound dumbbells, lie back on the bench, get as focused as I possibly can, and, while maintaining very strict form, I lower the weight, pausing for a moment at the bottom, and then I press it up while flexing my chest muscles. By the time I get to my eighth rep, my muscles are burning. By the time I get to the tenth rep, they are really burning. And the eleventh and twelfth reps are *very* challenging. That's level 9.

I set the 60-pound dumbbells down and immediately grab a pair of 40-pound dumbbells, lie back on the bench, and this time, instead of doing the dumbbell bench press, I do flyes. (See the Exercise Guide on page 135 for

bodyforlife.com   www.bodyforlife.com   www.bodyforlife.com   www.bodyforlife.com   www.bodyforlife.com   www.bodyforlife.c

detailed instructions and photos showing all the exercises I perform.) On this set, my muscles are already burning by the time I reach my fourth rep. I breathe in deeply as I slowly lower the weight, and I exhale as I lift the weight back up.

By about the seventh rep, my muscles are toast. By the ninth rep, I *really* want to set the weight down, but I know, from past experience, that this is exactly where I want to be. In my mind I think, "All right, Bill, three more reps. Don't quit now!"

By this point, the earth is moving—we've got a full-scale earthquake. I barely get the tenth rep—I'm at level 9 for sure. Once I start that eleventh rep, I immediately shift from training with my muscles to relying on my inner strength. (When you get there, you'll know what I'm talking about.)

Before the twelfth and final rep, I pause and ask, "How strong am I? How powerful is my inner strength?" Then, I reach deep down inside and go to level 10, as I overcome the resistance and succeed! (Already I've achieved a goal and hit a high point. Not a bad way to start a workout—not a bad way to start a day!)

I write down "10!" on my Progress Report and move on.

By now, I can really feel the blood rushing to the muscles in my chest. I'm also breathing pretty darn heavily. Speaking of breathing, when you're performing your weight-training exercises, you should inhale deeply, through your nose, during the eccentric (negative) part of the exercise, and breathe out deeply, through the mouth, during the concentric (positive) part of the exercise. For example, if you're doing the bench press, when you lower the weight, you should breathe in. When you press the weight up, breathe out.

I've got two minutes to catch my breath; then I begin my shoulder workout with the seated dumbbell press. I start with 30-pound dumbbells for 12 reps, wait one minute, then do my set of 10, then eight, then six. I follow my plan, which is shown on page 73.

Once I get the shoulder muscles primed, I reach for a high-point set, performing 12 reps of the seated dumbbell press, and then immediately going to my next exercise for shoulders called side raises, and I push it like crazy—trying to reach that level 10 intensity where I go above and beyond.

w.bodyforlife.com   www.bodyforlife.com   www.bodyforlife.com   www.bodyforlife.com   www.bodyforlife.com   www.bodyforli

On this set, after 12 reps, I feel I could have done one or two more. That's okay, I hit level 9. I simply make a note that the next time I do side raises, I'm going to try using 15-pound instead of 10-pound dumbbells. (It's so important to make notes and compare your plan to actual when you're doing these workouts. It's a constant process of fine-tuning, making slight modifications, and evolving.)

Remember, when you do the exercises, you might use more or less weight than I do. That doesn't matter. What does matter is what intensity level you reach compared to yourself.

I've got only 22 more minutes to finish, so I quickly move on to dumbbell rowing for the back muscles. After I finish my fifth set of that exercise, which I do for 12 reps with 70 pounds, I immediately go to an exercise called the dumbbell pullover. Remember, you can find photos and descriptions of all these exercises in the Exercise Guide on page 135. Be sure to follow the proper form, as it not only increases workout efficiency but also will prevent unnecessary muscle pulls and strains that can be caused by doing the exercise the wrong way. (You can also see video demonstrations of these exercises for free at www.bodyforlife.com.)

I'm telling you, by the time you get to these last few reps on that second set of 12, you've got to hone in your focus like a laser beam. You can't think about anything else. When I'm holding a 70-pound weight above my head, the last thing I'm concerned with is paperwork. It's survival of the fittest at this point. And you know what? It feels awesome. To truly be focused on only one thing—to be breathing, to have your blood circulating, to be moving and flexing—it's just awesome (and I try not to use that word too often).

By the way, if you do have the opportunity to exercise with someone—a friend, your spouse, your brother or sister, sometimes I even exercise with my mom—it's a terrific experience to share. It's so rare these days that people work together to accomplish goals—I mean really work together to do something positive with one another, for one another. It builds a powerful bond. When you do what you say you're going to do (show up for the workout) and get into it, you're also building mutual respect.

odyforlife.com   www.bodyforlife.com   www.bodyforlife.com   www.bodyforlife.com   www.bodyforlife.com   www.bodyforlife.c

The Training-for-LIFE Experience™
Daily Progress Report

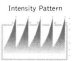
Intensity Pattern

Date: 5/4/99	
Day 1 of 84	
Upper Body Workout	

Planned Start Time: 6:05	Actual Start Time: 6:10
Planned End Time: 6:51	Actual End Time: 6:55
Time to Complete: 46 minutes	Total Time: 45 minutes

Upper Body Muscle Groups	Exercise	PLAN Reps	PLAN Weight (lbs)	PLAN Minutes Between Sets	PLAN Intensity Level	ACTUAL Reps	ACTUAL Weight (lbs)	ACTUAL Minutes Between Sets	ACTUAL Intensity Level
Chest	Dumbbell Bench Press	12	40	1	5	12	40	1	5
	Dumbbell Bench Press	10	50	1	6	10	50	1	6
	Dumbbell Bench Press	8	60	1	7	8	60	1	7
	Dumbbell Bench Press	6	70	1	8	6	70	1	8
High Point	Dumbbell Bench Press	12	60	0	9	12	60	0	9
	Dumbbell Flyes	12	40	2	10	12	40	2	10!
Shoulders	Seated Dumbbell Press	12	30	1	5	12	30	1	5
	Seated Dumbbell Press	10	40	1	6	10	40	1	6
	Seated Dumbbell Press	8	45	1	7	8	45	1	7
	Seated Dumbbell Press	6	50	1	8	6	50	1	8
High Point	Seated Dumbbell Press	12	45	0	9	12	45	0	9
	Side Raises	12	10	2	10	12	10	2	9
Back	Dumbbell Rows	12	50	1	5	12	50	1	5
	Dumbbell Rows	10	60	1	6	10	60	1	6
	Dumbbell Rows	8	70	1	7	8	70	1	7
	Dumbbell Rows	6	80	1	8	6	80	1	8
High Point	Dumbbell Rows	12	70	0	9	12	70	0	9
	Dumbbell Pullovers	12	70	2	10	12	70	2	9
Triceps	Seated Dumbbell Extensions	12	50	1	5	12	50	1	5
	Seated Dumbbell Extensions	10	60	1	6	10	60	1	6
	Seated Dumbbell Extensions	8	70	1	7	8	70	1	7
	Seated Dumbbell Extensions	6	80	1	8	6	80	1	8
High Point	Seated Dumbbell Extensions	12	70	0	9	12	70	0	9
	Lying Triceps Extensions	12	20	2	10	12	20	2	10

At this point, you should be 37 minutes into your upper body weight-training workout and have 9 minutes to go.

Biceps	Seated Dumbbell Curls	12	25	1	5	12	25	1	5
	Seated Dumbbell Curls	10	30	1	6	10	30	1	6
	Seated Dumbbell Curls	8	35	1	7	8	35	1	7
	Seated Dumbbell Curls	6	40	1	8	6	40	1	8
High Point	Seated Dumbbell Curls	12	35	0	9	12	35	0	9
	Standing Dumbbell Curls	12	30	–	10	12	30	–	9

NOTES

Need to go up to 15-pound dumbbells for side raises next time. I need to increase my

weight on dumbbell pullovers from 70 to 80 pounds and try harder. Great Workout!

.bodyforlife.com   www.bodyforlife.com   www.bodyforlife.com   www.bodyforlife.com   www.bodyforlife.com   www.bodyforlife

Anyway, after I finish my back workout, I move on to triceps, finish my sets there, then hit my favorite muscles—biceps.

I finish my last high-intensity set by performing 12 reps of standing dumbbell curls and check the clock—I brought it in right at 45 minutes.

Now, I sit down on the bench and take just three minutes to record my actual workout and compare it to my plan. I make a few notes such as, "I need to increase my weight on dumbbell pullovers next time from 70 to 80 pounds and try harder." And since I had a great workout, I write, "Great workout!" (Pretty simple, huh?)

My next weight-training workout is Wednesday. I exercise my leg muscles and abs that day using the same tools and techniques I used in the workout I just shared with you. I have included a copy of my lower body Daily Progress Report on page 77 for your review.

Now, let's take a look at the aerobic workout I perform on Tuesdays, Thursdays, and Saturdays.

Beginning the Day With a High Point

Tuesday morning I wake up at 6:30 A.M., drink two cups of water, put on my workout clothes, walk across the hall, and get on my stationary bike. No weight training today—just fat-burning aerobics.

I start pedaling at a steady pace—a level 5 on the Intensity Index. I do that for two minutes while I review my written goals. Then I start to increase the resistance on the stationary bike until I have to push a little harder. I maintain that pace for 60 seconds, then I increase the resistance so it requires a level 7 effort, then I go to level 8 and so on. I follow the plan on the opposite page.

If you've never performed aerobic exercise using intensity intervals, let me give you a heads up. It ain't easy! When I tell people I do 20 minutes of aerobic exercise, they scoff, "Is that all?"

"Yep," I tell them. "Here, you give a try." By the time they actually put the 20-Minute Aerobics Solution to the test, they're singing a different tune.

bodyforlife.com   www.bodyforlife.com   www.bodyforlife.com   www.bodyforlife.com   www.bodyforlife.com   www.bodyforlife.

The 20-Minute Aerobics Solution™
Daily Progress Report

Intensity Pattern

Date: 5/5/99	Planned Start Time: 6:40	Actual Start Time: 6:35
Day 2 of 84	Planned End Time: 7:00	Actual End Time: 6:55
Aerobic Workout	Time to Complete: 20 minutes	Total Time: 20 minutes

Exercise	PLAN		Exercise	ACTUAL	
	Minute by Minute	Intensity Level		Minute by Minute	Intensity Level
Stationary Bike	1	5	Stationary Bike	1	5
	2	5		2	5
	3	6		3	6
	4	7		4	7
	5	8		5	8
	6	9		6	9
	7	6		7	6
	8	7		8	7
	9	8		9	8
	10	9		10	9
	11	6		11	6
	12	7		12	7
	13	8		13	8
	14	9		14	9
	15	6		15	6
	16	7		16	7
	17	8		17	8
High Point	18	9	**High Point**	18	9
	19	10		19	9
	20	5		20	5

NOTES

Good workout. Quick but efficient.

Try harder next time!

This aerobic workout is a challenge. And, what I like most is that it is so darn efficient. (I like efficiency . . . a lot.)

Anyway, by the time I finish my 20-minute workout, I'm breathing heavily, my pulse rate is up, and I've worked up quite a sweat. I've also got the oxygen flowing to my brain. It's a great way to start the day.

Where I live, in the foothills of the Rocky Mountains, spring and summer mornings are absolutely glorious. (I don't use that word much either, but that's what they are, downright glorious!)

So I often do my 20-minute aerobic exercise outside during those months. There's something very powerful about being outdoors. In fact, it's downright unnatural for us to spend all our time under man-made light in a house, an office, a mall, or a grocery store. Now, granted, you don't want to spend so much time under the sun that you fry your skin—turning yourself into a human Gucci bag by age 42—but there's no question direct sunlight and fresh air invigorate the body and mind.

The workout is simple: I walk out the front door, click my stopwatch, and walk for two minutes. Then I gradually pick up the pace—walking, then jogging, then jogging faster, then walking again, and so on. I go through all four intensity interval cycles.

Make no mistake, I don't move like Terrell Davis when I "sprint"—my high-intensity run is not a "world-class event." But for me, it's a challenge. And I try to do a little better—to reach a little higher—each time. That's what matters.

I perform the 20-Minute Aerobics Solution three times a week and conduct my intense weight-training workouts three days a week, on alternate days. (See Your 12-Week Training-*for*-LIFE Schedule on page 78.) Through this integrated, high-intensity Program, my muscles receive all the "stimulation" they can handle. Doing any more than this would be a step backward, not forward.

After we complete our workouts, we must focus our attention on nutrition.

bodyforlife.com   www.bodyforlife.com   www.bodyforlife.com   www.bodyforlife.com   www.bodyforlife.com   www.bodyforlife

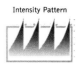
Date: 5/6/99	Planned Start Time: 6:30	Actual Start Time: 6:40
Day 3 of 84	Planned End Time: 7:12	Actual End Time: 7:25
Lower Body Workout	Time to Complete: 42 minutes	Total Time: 45 minutes

Lower Body Muscle Groups	Exercise	PLAN				ACTUAL			
		Reps	Weight (lbs)	Minutes Between Sets	Intensity Level	Reps	Weight (lbs)	Minutes Between Sets	Intensity Level
Quads	Leg Press	12	250	1	5	12	250	1	5
	Leg Press	10	300	1	6	10	300	1	6
	Leg Press	8	350	1	7	8	350	1	7
	Leg Press	6	400	1	8	6	400	1	8
High Point	Leg Press	12	350	0	9	12	350	0	9
	Leg Extensions	12	110	2	10	12	110	2	10
Hamstrings	Dumbbell Lunges	12	30	1	5	12	30	1	5
	Dumbbell Lunges	10	35	1	6	10	35	1	6
	Dumbbell Lunges	8	40	1	7	8	40	1	7
	Dumbbell Lunges	6	45	1	8	6	45	1	8
High Point	Dumbbell Lunges	12	40	0	9	12	40	0	9
	Lying Leg Curls	12	70	2	10	12	70	2	10
Calves	Standing Calf Raises	12	200	1	5	12	200	1	5
	Standing Calf Raises	10	250	1	6	10	250	1	6
	Standing Calf Raises	8	300	1	7	8	300	1	7
	Standing Calf Raises	6	350	1	8	6	350	1	8
High Point	Standing Calf Raises	12	300	0	9	12	300	0	9
	Seated Calf Raises	12	200	2	10	12	200	2	9
At this point, you should be 31 minutes into your lower body weight-training workout and have 11 minutes to go.									
Abs	Floor Crunches	12	-	1	5	12	-	1	5
	Floor Crunches	10	-	1	6	10	-	1	6
	Floor Crunches	8	-	1	7	8	-	1	7
	Floor Crunches	6	-	1	8	6	-	1	8
High Point	Floor Crunches	12	-	0	9	12	-	0	9
	Decline Sit-Ups	12	20	–	10	12	20	–	9

NOTES

Leg extensions felt fantastic—great burn.

Calves on fire. Go up to 220 next time for seated calf raises.

Try to go faster next time.

bodyforlife.com   www.bodyforlife.com   www.bodyforlife.com   www.bodyforlife.com   **www.bodyforlife.com**   www.bodyforlife

Your 12-Week Training-*for*-LIFE™ Schedule

	Monday	Tuesday	Wednesday	Thursday	Friday	Saturday	Sunday
Week 1	Day 1 Upper Body Weight Training	Day 2 20-Minute Aerobics Solution	Day 3 Lower Body Weight Training	Day 4 20-Minute Aerobics Solution	Day 5 Upper Body Weight Training	Day 6 20-Minute Aerobics Solution	Day 7 Free Day
Week 2	Day 8 Lower Body Weight Training	Day 9 20-Minute Aerobics Solution	Day 10 Upper Body Weight Training	Day 11 20-Minute Aerobics Solution	Day 12 Lower Body Weight Training	Day 13 20-Minute Aerobics Solution	Day 14 Free Day
Week 3	Day 15 Upper Body Weight Training	Day 16 20-Minute Aerobics Solution	Day 17 Lower Body Weight Training	Day 18 20-Minute Aerobics Solution	Day 19 Upper Body Weight Training	Day 20 20-Minute Aerobics Solution	Day 21 Free Day
Week 4	Day 22 Lower Body Weight Training	Day 23 20-Minute Aerobics Solution	Day 24 Upper Body Weight Training	Day 25 20-Minute Aerobics Solution	Day 26 Lower Body Weight Training	Day 27 20-Minute Aerobics Solution	Day 28 Free Day
Week 5	Day 29 Upper Body Weight Training	Day 30 20-Minute Aerobics Solution	Day 31 Lower Body Weight Training	Day 32 20-Minute Aerobics Solution	Day 33 Upper Body Weight Training	Day 34 20-Minute Aerobics Solution	Day 35 Free Day
Week 6	Day 36 Lower Body Weight Training	Day 37 20-Minute Aerobics Solution	Day 38 Upper Body Weight Training	Day 39 20-Minute Aerobics Solution	Day 40 Lower Body Weight Training	Day 41 20-Minute Aerobics Solution	Day 42 Free Day
Week 7	Day 43 Upper Body Weight Training	Day 44 20-Minute Aerobics Solution	Day 45 Lower Body Weight Training	Day 46 20-Minute Aerobics Solution	Day 47 Upper Body Weight Training	Day 48 20-Minute Aerobics Solution	Day 49 Free Day
Week 8	Day 50 Lower Body Weight Training	Day 51 20-Minute Aerobics Solution	Day 52 Upper Body Weight Training	Day 53 20-Minute Aerobics Solution	Day 54 Lower Body Weight Training	Day 55 20-Minute Aerobics Solution	Day 56 Free Day
Week 9	Day 57 Upper Body Weight Training	Day 58 20-Minute Aerobics Solution	Day 59 Lower Body Weight Training	Day 60 20-Minute Aerobics Solution	Day 61 Upper Body Weight Training	Day 62 20-Minute Aerobics Solution	Day 63 Free Day
Week 10	Day 64 Lower Body Weight Training	Day 65 20-Minute Aerobics Solution	Day 66 Upper Body Weight Training	Day 67 20-Minute Aerobics Solution	Day 68 Lower Body Weight Training	Day 69 20-Minute Aerobics Solution	Day 70 Free Day
Week 11	Day 71 Upper Body Weight Training	Day 72 20-Minute Aerobics Solution	Day 73 Lower Body Weight Training	Day 74 20-Minute Aerobics Solution	Day 75 Upper Body Weight Training	Day 76 20-Minute Aerobics Solution	Day 77 Free Day
Week 12	Day 78 Lower Body Weight Training	Day 79 20-Minute Aerobics Solution	Day 80 Upper Body Weight Training	Day 81 20-Minute Aerobics Solution	Day 82 Lower Body Weight Training	Day 83 20-Minute Aerobics Solution	Day 84 Free Day

Body-*for*-LIFE

Overview of The Training-*for*-LIFE Experience™ Principles

- Weight train, intensely, for no more than 46 minutes, three times per week: Monday, Wednesday, and Friday. Perform 20 minutes of aerobic exercise, first thing in the morning on an empty stomach, three times per week: Tuesday, Thursday, and Saturday. Take Sunday off—it's your free day.

- Alternate training the major muscles of the upper and lower body. For example, the first week, train upper body on Monday, lower body on Wednesday, and upper body on Friday. The second week, train lower body on Monday, upper body on Wednesday, and lower body on Friday. (See chart on the previous page.)

- Perform two exercises for each major muscle group of the upper body, which includes: chest, shoulders, back, triceps, and biceps; and for the lower body: quadriceps, hamstrings, and calves. Train the abdominal muscles after lower body.

- Select one exercise for each muscle group and conduct five sets, starting with a set of 12 reps, then increasing the weight and doing 10 reps, adding more weight and doing eight reps, adding more weight for six reps. Then reduce the weight, do 12 more reps, and immediately go to another set of 12 reps of another exercise for that muscle group.

- On all lifts, use a cadence of two seconds (say "I am building my Body-*for*-LIFE") to lower the weight and one second (say "Body-*for*-LIFE") to lift it, and "hold" in the top and bottom positions for a count of "one."

- For each muscle group, rest for one minute between the first four sets. Then complete the final two sets with no rest in between. Wait two minutes before moving on to your next muscle group. Complete this pattern five times for the upper body training experience and four times for the lower body training experience.

- Follow the Intensity Index pattern and push yourself to reach higher every week.

- Always plan your training beforehand. Plan what time you're going to exercise, which particular exercises you'll be doing, how much weight you'll be lifting, and how long it will take you to complete the session. Also, keep accurate records using the Training-*for*-LIFE Experience Daily Progress Reports on pages 175–187.

.bodyforlife.com   www.bodyforlife.com   www.bodyforlife.com   www.bodyforlife.com   www.bodyforlife.com   www.bodyforlife

The Eating-*for*-LIFE Method

—————————— Part V ——————————

*When you nourish your body with pure
energy, you transform from the inside out.*

Think about this for a moment: Within a year, virtually every cell which makes up your body right now will be gone.

No. That doesn't mean you'll be vaporized, nor does it mean Armageddon is at hand. The fact of the matter is your entire body is "re-created" every year. Out with the old, in with the new. Your skin, your muscles, even your organs are constantly degenerating and regenerating. It's going on *right now*. It's not something that's going to start tomorrow or a month from tomorrow or when you hit your next birthday.

As sure as you're reading the words on this page, this instant, your body is in that constant cycle of re-creation.

The pace of this process depends on your age. Somewhere around age 25, the natural process of "building up" that your body has undergone since birth crosses over to a process where degeneration occurs faster than regeneration. A similar process occurs with all living things. For example, a flower grows until it stops growing. Then it begins dying. This is natural.

But it's *not* inevitable. You see, unlike a flower, we *can* do something about this. We *can* adapt and evolve. We don't have to lose muscle, gain

81

fat, feel tired, give up, and give in as we age. If we choose, we can look and feel good, for life. We have the opportunity to re-create ourselves, *if* we decide to do it, and *if* we know how. (Don't worry, I'm gonna teach you just how to do that.)

Now, what do you think your body uses to re-create itself? Where does it get the raw materials to construct new skin cells, brain cells, muscle cells, bone cells, new blood, and even a new heart?

If you guessed "food," you're right. You see, in a very literal way, that old saying "You are what you eat" is true. And, even though most everyone has heard that saying time and time again, I've discovered that very few people *really* understand it.

Very few people are clear about the fundamentals of nutrition. It's just not something we usually learn in school or at work (unless you work for me) or from a coach or even a personal trainer.

In fact, many "experts" are *more* confused than the people they're supposed to be helping. Sometimes they don't know enough, and believe it or not, sometimes they know *too much*. By that, I mean they have read so many articles and textbooks, been to *so* many seminars, been exposed to so much information that they are overwhelmed—they suffer paralysis from analysis. They overthink the topic of nutrition and quite often are so caught up with the small stuff that they fail to clearly see the big picture.

What I see very clearly is that most people have no clue what they're doing to themselves with the food they normally eat. Nor are most people aware of how much better they could look *and* feel if they stopped feeding themselves accidentally and started *re-creating* themselves intentionally.

The good news is, it doesn't have to be complicated. What I've taught thousands of people—and what you are about to learn—isn't rocket science. In fact, once you get the hang of it, it's downright simple. Once you discover the right method of feeding your body, you'll never have to relearn it. It's kinda like learning how to drive a car—it's a bit intimidating at first, but with a little practice, you'll be "up to speed."

bodyforlife.com   www.bodyforlife.com   www.bodyforlife.com   www.bodyforlife.com   www.bodyforlife.com   www.bodyforlife

Remember, quality nutrition is just as important as the exercise techniques you read about in the previous section. (Exercise is the *spark*. Nutrition is the *fuel*. Without *both*, there can be no flame—no results.) So as soon as you start exercising intensely, you must begin eating the *right* way; you must start consistently feeding your body what it *needs* to re-create itself, so you can enjoy rapid and rewarding progress. With that in mind, here's a list of quality, nutrient-rich foods I recommend:

Eating-*for*-LIFE *Authorized* Foods

Proteins	Carbohydrates	Vegetables
chicken breast	baked potato	broccoli
turkey breast	sweet potato	asparagus
lean ground turkey	yam	lettuce
swordfish	squash	carrots
orange roughy	pumpkin	cauliflower
haddock	steamed brown rice	green beans
salmon	steamed wild rice	green peppers
tuna	pasta	mushrooms
crab	oatmeal	spinach
lobster	barley	tomato
shrimp	beans	peas
top round steak	corn	brussels sprouts
top sirloin steak	strawberries	artichoke
lean ground beef	melon	cabbage
buffalo	apple	celery
lean ham	orange	zucchini
egg whites or substitutes	fat-free yogurt	cucumber
low-fat cottage cheese	whole-wheat bread	onion

Choose a portion of protein and carbohydrates from each column to make a meal. Add a serving of vegetables to at least two of your daily meals.

.bodyforlife.com   www.bodyforlife.com   www.bodyforlife.com   www.bodyforlife.com   www.**bodyforlife.com**   www.bodyforlife

I'm sure you saw plenty of the foods you enjoy eating on the chart on the previous page. Simply choose one portion from each column in any combination. For example: grilled chicken (protein), steamed brown rice (carbohydrate), and spinach (vegetable). There are dozens of different meals you can prepare from the authorized foods list. I'll show you some more examples later in this section, but first, let's take a closer look at some of the foods that will help nourish our bodies and enrich our lives.

Quality Proteins

Poultry (Chicken and Turkey)

Chicken and turkey breasts are excellent choices of whole-food proteins. They're low in fat (once you get rid of the skin and bake or grill them instead of frying them), high in protein, and are available practically anywhere, anytime. You can roast, broil, grill, or sauté them.

You can also buy poultry in ground form and make meat loaf, tacos, or hamburgers out of it. One note of caution, though: If you buy ground chicken or turkey from the grocery store or butcher, make sure it's ground *breast* meat. Most ground poultry and deli meats have dark meat in them and possibly some pieces of skin or organ meat and other "stuff" that I haven't authorized and you don't wanna know about.

Fish and Shellfish

Seafood is another great protein food. Good choices of fish include salmon, tuna, cod, haddock, halibut, perch, sea bass, snapper, and swordfish. Shellfish, like crab and lobster, are also high in protein and low in fat. You can't go wrong with these choices, as long as you bake or grill the fish—don't deep fry it or cover it with butter or a high-fat sauce.

bodyforlife.com   www.bodyforlife.com   www.bodyforlife.com   www.bodyforlife.com   www.bodyforlife.com   www.bodyforlife

Red Meat (Beef, Buffalo, Venison)

Red meat is bad for you—it's a guilty pleasure, full of fat and cholesterol, right? Well, not really. Lean meat is high in protein and only about seven percent fat. (Choose the top round cut, top sirloin, shank, round, flank, or chuck to keep the saturated fat low.)

Although coronary artery disease continues to be the leading cause of death in America, the cholesterol found in lean red meat is *not* to blame. Lean beef (top round steak, 71 mg), chicken (breast, skinned, 72 mg), and fish (flounder, 58 mg) are very close in cholesterol content. The fact is, it's the overconsumption of saturated fat and the lack of proper exercise that contribute most to heart disease.

Low-Fat Cottage Cheese

Of all the protein foods you can choose, low-fat cottage cheese *may* be the best. You see, it's rich with amino acids, one of them being glutamine, which helps support muscle metabolism. And it's also a complete protein, which means it contains all the amino acids necessary to build new muscle, as well as support the body's other protein requirements.

Another advantage low-fat cottage cheese has over some of our other protein choices is that you don't have to cook it: You can take it with you in a cooler or keep some in your refrigerator. It's always there when you need it.

Egg Whites and Egg Substitutes

Packed with protein, low in calories, zero cholesterol, and no fat—egg whites get an A+. They have long been the favorite source of protein for athletes and are now being consumed daily by many people who are following my Body-*for*-LIFE Program.

One cautionary note, though. Never eat your egg whites raw or undercooked, or you may be at risk for salmonella poisoning. In order to kill any salmonella bacteria that may be on or in the egg, you have to boil the egg

w.bodyforlife.com   www.bodyforlife.com   www.bodyforlife.com   www.bodyforlife.com   www.bodyforlife.com   www.bodyforlif

for at least seven minutes, poach it for at least five minutes, or fry it for at least three minutes per side. Omelets and scrambled eggs should be cooked until dry.

The easiest and least expensive way to eat egg whites is to simply crack open an egg and remove the yolk. However, because you should not eat raw eggs, there are times when egg substitutes are a better choice. I like Egg Beaters better than egg whites, especially for making omelets.

Quality Carbohydrates

Potato

If I had to pick my favorite carbohydrate food, potatoes would be it. They're conveniently "nature made" in portion sizes—all you do is pick one that is approximately the size of your clenched fist. (See how simple that is?)

Potatoes go well with almost any protein portion, and they're portable, refrigeratable, and, contrary to popular belief, they taste great even without butter and sour cream. You can top them with a spoonful of salsa, ketchup, steak sauce—they're even great plain.

Brown Rice

Steamed brown rice (and by steamed, I mean not boiled with butter) is my second favorite carbohydrate choice.

The main difference between brown and white rice is how they've been processed. This changes the way the body uses the carbohydrates. Remember food is our bodies' source of fuel. And, brown rice burns much slower than white rice. This means you will have more energy for a longer period of time when you eat brown rice. The main thing you need to remember is that a portion of steamed brown rice combined with a portion of a quality protein and a vegetable is a meal.

odyforlife.com   www.bodyforlife.com   www.bodyforlife.com   www.bodyforlife.com   www.bodyforlife.com   www.bodyforlife.c

Oatmeal

Oatmeal is the favorite carbohydrate portion among many people who are following the Body-*for*-LIFE Program. It's easy to make, nutritious, inexpensive, and it tastes good. (I sprinkle NutraSweet and cinnamon on mine.)

A word of caution—there are a lot of high-sugar instant oatmeals you would be better off avoiding, especially when good old-fashioned Quaker Oats are the better choice.

Barley

Although it's not my favorite, barley may be the best carbohydrate food there is. Barley comes in flake or pearl form. Both can be cooked and eaten as a hot cereal. The most nutritious form of barley and, ironically, the hardest to find, is hulled barley. Even though it's rarely found in supermarkets, it can usually be picked up at the local health-food store.

Although barley is often used in soups, you can also use it to make hot cereal. It's a little bland, but the flavor can easily be improved by adding some NutraSweet and cinnamon.

Pasta

Spaghetti, linguini, macaroni . . . whatever you call it, pasta is a good low-fat source of carbohydrates. The key to making pasta work for you on this Program is to recognize the difference between a plateful and a portion. Many people think that because pasta is low in fat, they can eat all they want.

Also, no Alfredo sauce, butter, or cheese. When I do eat pasta, I usually eat it plain or just squeeze lemon over it. Nice and simple and clean.

Sweet Potatoes or Yams

Because of its sweetness, many people assume the sweet potato is higher in calories than a regular potato. Not so. Because of an enzyme in the potato that converts starches into sugars, the vegetable tastes very sweet. It actually

v.bodyforlife.com   www.bodyforlife.com   www.bodyforlife.com   www.bodyforlife.com   www.bodyforlife.com   www.bodyforli

has no more calories than a regular potato. Baking, boiling, or microwaving are the best ways to prepare them; in fact, they can be cooked the same way as regular potatoes.

Make sure when you bring them home from the grocery store that you don't put them in the refrigerator, where they may become hard and bitter tasting. Instead, store them in a cool, dry place where they will keep for about a month. If they're stored at room temperature on a kitchen counter, they'll keep for only about a week.

Yogurt

Yogurt qualifies as a carbohydrate choice on our Program, which means, of course, it should be combined with a portion of protein to make a meal. Sometimes I mix nonfat yogurt and cottage cheese for a quick and easy mid-morning or evening meal. However, I'm not talking about frozen yogurt, which is too high in sugar to make my authorized list. Also remember that eating yogurt by itself is not a meal: You've got to combine it with protein.

Fruit

Here's another carbohydrate that nature has pre-portioned for us. An apple, an orange, a peach, a banana: They're all portions of carbohydrates, and they're rich with nutrients, generally portable, and when you simply combine them with a portion of protein, you've got a meal.

Whole-Wheat Bread

Usually, when people start the Body-for-LIFE Program, I try to wean them off of bread, crackers, cookies, and other carbohydrate foods that they've been overdosing on, and, although I'm reluctant to "authorize" bread, I do so under the condition that it be whole-wheat bread and that you understand that a portion of bread generally, unless you've got one big ol' hand, is only two slices of bread or one whole-wheat tortilla. Therefore, authorized meals may include a couple of my favorites, a grilled-chicken sandwich or chicken pita.

bodyforlife.com   www.bodyforlife.com   www.bodyforlife.com   www.bodyforlife.com   www.bodyforlife.com   www.bodyforlife.c

Vegetables

High-nutrient, healthy foods that are not a significant source of protein or carbohydrates, but which should be included with at least two of your daily meals include: spinach, broccoli, tomatoes, carrots, lettuce, cauliflower, celery, cucumbers, green beans, squash, asparagus, cabbage, and mushrooms.

These vegetables are not only low in calories but are high in fiber and/or contain antioxidants (which have been shown in scientific studies to help prevent cancer), and they're just plain good for you, if they're not cooked in butter, covered with cheese, or deep-fat fried. You can buy them fresh or frozen and serve them lightly steamed or raw.

Healthy Fats

Despite popular belief, not all fats are bad: Saturated fats are the enemy. Unsaturated fats, in moderate amounts, can actually be good for you. For example, one of the reasons fish is such a healthy food is because it contains essential fatty acids (often called EFAs), which can actually help your body burn fat more efficiently and protect you from certain diseases.

There's a general rule for knowing which fats are okay and which ones are not okay: If it is solid at room temperature, like butter, margarine, or shortening, it's bad news. (A couple of exceptions to that rule are palm oil and coconut oil—they're both saturated fats that are primarily stored as body fat and cause an increase in cholesterol.)

Good fats include safflower oil, sesame oil, canola oil, and the fat in avocados. Now, that doesn't mean you need a portion of any of these fats. Just a tablespoon a day can provide your body with the essential fatty acids it needs. For example, you can mix a tablespoon of safflower oil with vinegar and use it as salad dressing. And, if you eat fish, especially salmon, at least three times a week, chances are you're getting the essential fatty acids you need.

.bodyforlife.com   www.bodyforlife.com   www.bodyforlife.com   www.bodyforlife.com   www.bodyforlife.com   www.bodyforlife

The Performance Nutrition Advantage™

Although eating six times a day might seem expensive and time consuming, I've discovered a method which saves time and money, while taking the guesswork out of "eating right." It involves using a high-tech nutrition shake that was designed by my company, Experimental and Applied Sciences (EAS). It's called Myoplex, and it's already helped literally tens of thousands of people complete their Program. In fact, virtually every person who finished our last 12-week Transformation Challenge used Myoplex.

I call Myoplex The Performance Nutrition Advantage because it offers an "extra edge" for so many people who accept my challenge to put the Body-*for*-LIFE Program to the test but aren't used to eating frequent, high-nutrient meals, day in and day out.

Myoplex is so simple—it's a powder you just mix with water in a shaker or blender. In less than a minute, you can create a "super shake" (it's like a nutritious milk shake) that contains a precise blend of nutrients your body needs to maintain proper health and recover quickly from your strenuous workouts.

Think of it this way: Let's say you took a grocery cart full of healthy whole foods such as lean meat, fruits, vegetables, and dairy products and extracted the valuable nutrients—the good things the body needs—and put them in one place; and took all the leftover junk—the excess calories and saturated fat—and got rid of it.

Then, if you took all of the good stuff and combined it in precise ratios, what you would have is a custom-designed food—a precise formula that offers the positive biochemical effects of food without the negative. That's what Myoplex is: A high-tech fast food that has been scientifically designed to "starve" fat while *feeding* your muscles.

I use Myoplex every day and have for the past four years. Without the advantage it offers, I don't believe I would have been able to stick with this nutrition method which has helped me stay in top shape year after year. Plus, I'm not the type that likes to take handfuls of vitamin pills and whatnot. I'm too

bodyforlife.com   www.bodyforlife.com   www.bodyforlife.com   www.bodyforlife.com   www.bodyforlife.com   www.bodyforlife.

busy for that, and my guess is that you are, too. That's another reason I use Myoplex—three servings a day provide my body with 150 percent of the recommended daily allowance of 29 essential vitamins and minerals. Not only that, each shake contains more quality protein than a chicken breast, as much energy-rich carbohydrates as a portion of brown rice, and is very low in fat.

Now, I'm not saying you can't get good results with just regular food. That is possible, especially if you have time to shop for and prepare six quality whole-food meals day in and day out. However, many of the people I coach, especially athletes like John Elway, Mike Piazza, Terrell Davis, as well as businessmen, working mothers, and even soldiers, just don't have time to eat six whole-food meals a day. So for them, Myoplex is a solution—an advantage that makes following the Eating-*for*-LIFE Method much more practical. It may offer benefits for you as well. (If you would like more information about Myoplex, call EAS at 1-800-297-9776 [Dept. #17] or visit www.eas.com.)

Plan Your Grocery Shopping

Another thing you can do to help adopt this new pattern of eating—of *intentionally* feeding your body the nutrients it needs to re-create itself—is to make sure your cupboards and refrigerator are stocked with authorized foods. I'll say it yet again: If you fail to plan, you're planning to fail. By that, I mean, if you don't plan to have these foods available when and where you need them, it could be difficult to stick with the Program. Planning your meals starts by making a list before you go to the grocery store. Stock up only on quality sources of protein, carbohydrates, and vegetables.

Your Free Day

Six days a week, you need to follow the eating guidelines I've been telling you about in this section. And on the seventh day? Forget about them.

I mean forget them all. Eat whatever you want. If you want to have blueberry pancakes with syrup for breakfast or a cinnamon roll with coffee or milk,

.bodyforlife.com   www.bodyforlife.com   www.bodyforlife.com   www.bodyforlife.com   www.bodyforlife.com   www.bodyforlife

that's fine. If you want a Big Mac or two for lunch, go for it. If you want a thick pizza with everything on it for dinner, be my guest. If you want apple pie and ice cream for dessert, that's okay with me.

There is actually a physiological reason to purposely overeat once a week—it may help convince your body that it is not starving. Giving yourself a good feed once a week may calm that thousand-year-old encoded alarm inside your brain that goes off every time you begin to burn stored body fat for fuel.

But beyond the biological reasons, there are psychological benefits to the free day that are even greater, at least as far as I'm concerned. One of the many things I've learned from working with people hands-on over the years, not just through a laboratory, not just through reading what scientific studies say, is that as soon as you say to someone, "Okay, you're looking at 12 weeks with absolutely no spaghetti and meatballs, no pizza, no ice cream, not even a jelly bean," you've invaded that person's circle of choice—you've taken away one of his or her perceived rights.

Most people need to know they have some degree of autonomy, that they are allowed to make certain decisions for themselves. They're willing to draw some lines and create a framework, a structure, as long as there's an element of freedom that remains.

You don't want to set yourself up for failure. You don't want to create standards you can't meet. If you say, "I'm not going to eat anything I shouldn't for the next 12 weeks," you've set yourself up for disappointment. That's like Michael Jordan going into a game and saying, "I'm not going to miss a shot."

No one wants to play a game he or she can't win. That's why I've built the free day into the Body-*for*-LIFE Program. I can't describe the difference this makes in a person's ability to stay with the Program. By having one day completely to yourself, you are downright eager to get into the next week's positive patterns of action.

I've also discovered that this free day serves the purpose of reminding you of what you used to feel like when every day was free day. It can keep

bodyforlife.com   www.bodyforlife.com   www.bodyforlife.com   www.bodyforlife.com   www.bodyforlife.com   www.bodyforlife.

you in touch with what you're trying to get away from—the sluggishness, indigestion, and energy drain created by overeating and infrequent eating.

As far as when you should have your free day, that's up to you. Some set aside every Sunday to eat whatever they want. Other times, you might want to go with the flow, adjusting your day to the circumstances of that week. Let's say you have a special occasion coming up and you know you're going to be eating in a social environment and don't want to worry about rules. That's fine. Plan ahead and make that your free day for the week.

As I mentioned before, I like to eat pizza every now and then. And I like my mom's chicken enchiladas. So that free day has been one of the keys to my maintaining this approach for a lifetime. The Body-*for*-LIFE Program is just that—for life. It's not something I do for just a certain amount of time. It's the way I live. And it will be for you as well, by the time the next 12 weeks are over.

And here's a little tip: The end of your free day is a great time to do your grocery shopping for the upcoming week. Your hunger will be more than satisfied, so the urge to buy tempting but inappropriate or unhealthy foods will be minimized.

Food for Change

Don't fall for the common misconception that healthy, high-nutrient meals have to be bland and boring—that's just not the case. The meals I eat taste good to me and are relatively simple to prepare. And most importantly, they provide my body with the quality nutrition I need. What follows is a sample of a few typical days on the Eating-*for*-LIFE Method. I've also included one of my Daily Progress Reports to show you how I keep track of, and compare, my plan-to-actual food and water intake.

.bodyforlife.com   www.bodyforlife.com   www.bodyforlife.com   www.bodyforlife.com   www.bodyforlife.com   www.bodyforlife

Six Monday Meals (Examples)

Breakfast: Ultra-Fast Egg-White Omelet

Beat four egg whites and one whole egg (or use Egg Beaters) with two tablespoons of skim milk. Toss eggs in a skillet lightly coated with a nonfat cooking spray, like Pam. Serve with two pieces of whole-wheat toast, and you've got a quality portion of protein and carbohydrates. Now drink two cups of ice water, and you're set.

Midmorning: Chocolate Nutrition Shake

Mix one serving of chocolate Myoplex with 12 to 16 ounces of cold water in a blender. Add three ice cubes. Blend at high speed for 45 seconds and serve.

Lunch: Tuna Salad

Drain a can of water-packed tuna. Then place tuna in a bowl and mix in one tablespoon of fat-free mayonnaise, one teaspoon of dill pickle relish, and juice from a lemon slice. Pile tuna on top of lettuce, and serve with a portion of fruit and two cups of ice water for a complete meal.

Midafternoon: Key Lime Pie Nutrition Shake

Mix one serving of a vanilla Myoplex according to directions. Then add two tablespoons of frozen limeaid concentrate and three ice cubes. Blend at high speed for 45 seconds and serve.

Dinner: Baked Turkey With Cranberry Sauce

Thinly slice a baked turkey breast. Microwave one tablespoon of cranberry sauce in a small bowl until warm (about 30 seconds). Pour cranberry sauce over turkey breast. Serve with a portion of steamed brown rice and broccoli along with two cups of ice water.

Late Evening: Chocolate-Berry Nutrition Shake

Mix one serving of a chocolate Myoplex according to directions. Then, add four frozen strawberries. Blend on high speed for 45 seconds and serve.

bodyforlife.com   www.bodyforlife.com   www.bodyforlife.com   www.bodyforlife.com   www.bodyforlife.com   www.bodyforlife.

Six Tuesday Meals

Breakfast: Zesty Breakfast Burrito

Fill a small whole-wheat tortilla with four scrambled egg whites or Egg Beaters. Add one tablespoon of salsa, half a tablespoon of low-fat shredded cheddar cheese, and one tablespoon of low-fat sour cream. Roll and serve along with a tall glass of ice water.

Midmorning: Chocolate-Mint Nutrition Shake

Mix one serving of a chocolate Myoplex according to directions. Then add three drops of peppermint extract and three ice cubes. Blend at high speed for 45 seconds and serve.

Lunch: Grilled Chicken Soup

In a small sauce pan, mix one can of chicken broth; a sliced, grilled chicken breast; a portion of cooked barley; and a handful of your favorite mixed vegetables. (The frozen ones are not only convenient, they're just as nutritious as fresh vegetables.) Warm over medium heat for five minutes and serve with two cups of ice water or iced tea.

Midafternoon: Strawberry-Frost Nutrition Shake

Mix one serving of strawberry Myoplex according to directions. Add three ice cubes. Blend at high speed for 45 seconds and serve.

Dinner: Grilled Salmon and Potato

Prepare a salmon steak by squeezing fresh lemon juice over it. Grill salmon for 10 to 15 minutes or until it flakes easily when tested with a fork. Serve with a baked potato, steamed spinach, and ice water.

Late Evening: Cinnamon Roll Supreme Nutrition Shake

Mix one serving of a vanilla Myoplex powder according to directions. Then add one half teaspoon ground cinnamon, one teaspoon fat-free Butter Buds, and three ice cubes. Blend at high speed for 45 seconds and serve.

bodyforlife.com   www.bodyforlife.com   www.bodyforlife.com   www.bodyforlife.com   **www.bodyforlife.com**   www.bodyforlife

Six Wednesday Meals (Examples)

Breakfast: Orange-Cream Nutrition Shake

Mix one serving of vanilla Myoplex according to directions. Add one half fresh orange plus three ice cubes. Blend on high speed for 45 seconds and serve.

Midmorning: Cottage Cheese and Yogurt

Mix a portion of cottage cheese with a portion of fat-free, sugar-free yogurt (I like blueberry Yoplait) for a nutrient-rich, quick, and easy meal. Don't forget to drink your water—two cups.

Lunch: Lemon-Lime Chicken and Potato

Smother a grilled, skinless chicken breast with freshly squeezed lemon and lime juices. Microwave a plain potato, and serve it with fresh carrots and a tall glass of iced tea.

Midafternoon: Rich Vanilla Nutrition Shake

Blend one serving of vanilla Myoplex with cold water and serve.

Dinner: Southwestern Steak and Rice

Place steak in a glass baking dish and pierce the meat with a knife or fork. Squeeze the juice from half a lime over the meat and sprinkle with pepper and garlic powder. Bake at 350° F until it's cooked to your liking. Then slice and serve with steamed brown rice covered with salsa, and salad with one tablespoon of safflower oil. If you wish, a glass of red wine can be added.

Late Evening: Double Chocolate Nutrition Shake

Blend one serving of a chocolate Myoplex with water. Add one serving of fat-free, sugar-free hot cocoa mix and three ice cubes. Blend at high speed for 45 seconds and serve.

bodyforlife.com   www.bodyforlife.com   www.bodyforlife.com   www.bodyforlife.com   www.bodyforlife.com   www.bodyforlife

The Eating-*for*-LIFE Method
Daily Progress Report

Date: 5/4/99	Day 1 of 84

Total portions of protein: 6	Total portions of protein: 6
Total portions of carbs: 6	Total portions of carbs: 6
Total cups of water: 10	Total cups of water: 11

PLAN		ACTUAL	
Meal 1	Breakfast burrito	**Meal 1**	Breakfast burrito
8:00 ☑a.m. ☐p.m.	2 cups water	7:50 ☑a.m. ☐p.m.	2 cups water
Meal 2	Chocolate Myoplex shake	**Meal 2**	Chocolate Myoplex shake
10:00 ☑a.m. ☐p.m.	made with 2 cups water	10:15 ☑a.m. ☐p.m.	made with 2 cups water
Meal 3	Chicken sandwich	**Meal 3**	Chicken sandwich
12:00 ☐a.m. ☑p.m.	1 cup water	12:00 ☐a.m. ☑p.m.	2 cups water
Meal 4	Strawberry Myoplex shake	**Meal 4**	Strawberry Myoplex shake
3:00 ☐a.m. ☑p.m.	made with 2 cups water	3:15 ☐a.m. ☑p.m.	made with 2 cups water
Meal 5	Grilled salmon	**Meal 5**	Grilled salmon
6:00 ☐a.m. ☑p.m.	Potato	6:10 ☐a.m. ☑p.m.	Potato
	Salad		Salad
	2 cups water		2 cups water
Meal 6	Myoplex pudding	**Meal 6**	Myoplex pudding
9:00 ☐a.m. ☑p.m.	1 cup water	9:15 ☐a.m. ☑p.m.	1 cup water

NOTES

I feel great! High energy all day.

I wasn't hungry at all.

Overview of The Eating-*for*-LIFE Method Principles

- Eat six small meals a day, one every two to three hours.

- Eat a portion of protein and carbohydrates with each meal.

- Add a portion of vegetables to at least two meals daily.

- A portion is the amount of an authorized food approximately the size of the palm of your hand or your clenched fist.

- Consume one tablespoon of unsaturated oil daily *or* three portions of salmon per week.

- Drink at least 10 cups of water a day.

- Use performance-nutrition shakes if necessary to make sure you're consuming optimal levels of required nutrients.

- Plan your meals in advance, and record what you eat, using the Eating-*for*-LIFE Method Daily Progress Reports on pages 175–187.

- Plan your grocery list.

- Once a week, on your free day, eat *whatever* you want.

bodyforlife.com   www.bodyforlife.com   www.bodyforlife.com   www.bodyforlife.com   www.bodyforlife.com   www.bodyforlife

Staying on Course

———————— Part VI ————————

Life, the ultimate challenge, is not a race to the finish but rather a process of continual growth.

Let's talk a little basic physics—getting an object at rest to begin moving requires far more energy than it does to keep it moving. Think of a rocket: 90 percent of the power is spent on the initial thrust—on getting the blasted thing into the air. The remaining 10 percent is all that's needed to keep it going. However, if that rocket strays off course, it requires considerable energy to get it back on track, and, if it gets too far off course, it will not complete its mission, and all the energy expended to lift it out of the gravitational pull of the earth is for naught.

In a way, the same applies to transforming our bodies. In fact, when shifting or changing *any* aspect of our lives, it's the act of getting started that is, by far, the most challenging stage of the process—a process which you've already begun. You're already generating considerable momentum. And if you keep it going, you will soon be experiencing impressive results. *Unless . . .* you stray off course. But, all too often, that's what *does* happen—people are going along great, then they quit. I don't want that to happen. Neither do you.

So now what I'm going to share with you are powerful solutions to challenges which lie ahead—challenges that can be transformed into energy to fuel your ascent instead of slowing you down, or worse yet, stopping you altogether.

99

Transform Adversity Into Energy

Picture this: For the first time in a long time, or perhaps the first time ever, all aspects of your life are coming together. You've successfully transformed your patterns of action, and you're moving forward in the direction of your goals.

You're looking better each week. That stubborn fat is finally melting away. In its place, muscle is forming. You're getting stronger, healthier. You're well on your way to a new and better life. You feel unstoppable until . . . the "unexpected" happens. Adversity strikes. Something goes wrong. You're blindsided by a bad hit.

These "hits" can come from any direction. It might be an injury that makes it difficult to exercise. It might be the loss of your job or a failed business venture, an illness, the end of a relationship, or worst of all, a personal tragedy.

The fact is, adversity hits all of us, and not just "once in a blue moon." No one is exempt. When trouble, in whatever form, strikes, it can bring your progress to a screeching halt. It can destroy your momentum, cripple your self-confidence, and send you into a tailspin—a situation where one thing after another, after another just doesn't go your way.

There's no training system, supplement, or "miracle pill" that can make you immune to adversity. But does that mean there's nothing you can do about it?

Yes and no.

You can't always prevent ill fortune, especially due to forces and circumstances beyond your control. But what you can do is expect adversity as an inevitable part of life. In fact, you must expect trouble in order to properly deal with it. Remember, it's not a matter of if it comes your way; it's a matter of when and how severely it strikes your life.

We must all accept that ill fortune is an inevitable part of life, and it is because of, not in spite of, misfortune that we grow. You see, our character will never be fully tested until things are not going our way. Those who have the

odyforlife.com   www.bodyforlife.com   www.bodyforlife.com   www.bodyforlife.com   www.bodyforlife.com   www.bodyforlife.c

courage to succeed *in spite of* adversity become an inspiration. They contribute value to the lives of others. They make a difference.

So, during the course of your 12-week Program, whenever you encounter adversity—whenever something comes up that you believe might prevent you from finishing your Program and successfully transforming your body and life—*immediately* ask yourself, "What can I do to turn this negative into a positive? How can I make this work *for me* rather than against me?"

When you approach obstacles this way, you will experience an immediate boost in energy and confidence (both of which you will need to complete your 12-week Program). And by practicing this skill—by learning how to transform obstacles into advantages—by attacking challenges head on—you will not only continue to move forward, you will gain the *inner strength* to deal with anything life brings your way.

When you look at adversity this way, you will realize misfortune is a bridge, not a barricade, to greater achievements. It can represent the opening of doors, not the closing of them. When adversity strikes, don't let it stop you. Promise yourself in advance you will transform that negative into a positive. That's not just the right way to handle it, it's the only way.

Honor Self-Promises

When you begin your 12-week Body-*for*-LIFE Program, you must promise yourself you will finish what you start, *no matter what*. That vow, although it might be easy to break, is by far one of the most important ones to honor. You see, the very essence of confidence is self-trust. Would you trust anyone who repeatedly lied to you? Someone who broke the rules of the game, again and again? Of course you wouldn't. So, if you've developed a pattern of not honoring self-promises, this is a great time to make a change. If you can't honor, trust, and depend on your own word, well . . . that may be the root of a lot of the challenges in your life—a lot more than you realize.

.bodyforlife.com   www.bodyforlife.com   www.bodyforlife.com   www.bodyforlife.com   www.bodyforlife.com   www.bodyforlife

This is a critical—and eye-opening—issue for each of us to face.

Most people have a very hard time answering the simple question, "Do I keep my word to myself?" Or, I should say, they have a hard time answering it *honestly*.

The thing about lying to ourselves is we never, ever get away with it. On the surface, we may fool our minds into ignoring or not admitting what we're doing, but deep down, in the place where all truth resides for each of us, in the place where we know and see ourselves as we really are—in that place, we are causing pain and damage every time we're not totally honest with ourselves.

For example, when you know darn well, deep down inside, that you should be doing something and you're not, like exercising regularly, like eating right, like finishing your 12-week Program, you're lying to yourself. Do it often enough, and your self-trust—your confidence—will fade away. Into that emptiness will seep uncertainty, anxiety, and anger.

It doesn't have to be like that though. No matter how long it has been like that, it doesn't have to stay that way. Contrary to what many people think, it's a lot easier to keep the promises we make to ourselves than it is to break them.

Keeping those promises unleashes enormous energy and potential. That potential emptiness created by self-deception will become filled with strength, certainty—and, yes, confidence—if you honor self-promises. (We've all heard the phrase, "The truth shall set you free." Well, nowhere is that more true than when we apply it to our relationship with ourselves.)

If you've gotten this far on these pages, you're already well into the process. You've already promised yourself you will not quit. This is not something to take lightly. This promise must be treated as earnestly as a vow you make to your spouse. Or to your child. Or to your boss or coach. Approach it with that feeling, and you will keep it. And when you succeed, you will *feel* the transformation inside even more than others see it on the outside. That, by the way, is a promise.

bodyforlife.com   www.bodyforlife.com   www.bodyforlife.com   www.bodyforlife.com   www.bodyforlife.com   www.bodyforlife.

Harness the Power of Positive Pressure

I've noticed that many people who begin their transformations with full force end up losing their drive after a few weeks. One way I help them overcome that setback is to teach them how to harness the power of positive pressure.

My observation is this: Most people in America have been conditioned (that means someone or some system has taught them) to believe they should "coast" through life as much as possible—they should avoid "pressure situations" and gravitate toward circumstances where no one is demanding anything from them. This is not good. It's not good at all, especially if you've decided to change your body and life. You see, contrary to popular belief, deep down inside, you want pressure; in fact, you need pressure to feel excited and passionate about life.

Real-life examples of people performing heroically under pressure can be seen everywhere: the fireman who rescues a child from a burning building, without a moment to spare; the quarterback who scores the winning touchdown, with time running out on the clock; the doctor who saves a dying patient's life.

The fact of the matter is, we are all capable of so much more than we might believe we are, but our ultimate potential is often smothered by what society teaches us—that pressure is a bad thing, that it hurts rather than helps our efforts to improve and become successful. Eventually, after years of conditioning, most people see pressure as an obstacle, not the powerful, driving force it really is.

You see, the truth of the matter is that it's through pressure or "stress" that we evolve—that we grow.

Think about it: The fundamental principle of building a stronger body is the process of overcoming stress, or "resistance." We force our muscles to work, and this effort in turn forces our muscles to adapt. If we put no pressure at all on those muscles, if we present them with no resistance whatsoever, what happens? They atrophy. They dissipate. They weaken.

w.bodyforlife.com   www.bodyforlife.com   www.bodyforlife.com   www.bodyforlife.com   **www.bodyforlife.com**   www.bodyforli

The same equation applies to our growth in the areas of our careers, our relationships, and our knowledge. It is only through the right amount of pressure that we continue to move beyond the level of mere existence or "comfort."

To harness the power of positive pressure, start with regularly subjecting your muscles to a healthy dose of stress by working out. Then, invite other challenges back into your life. Rather than run from pressure situations, or pretend they don't exist, face them. Seek them out. In doing so, you'll find that positive pressure brings out your best. You'll be raising it to a new, higher level.

And that, in every aspect of our lives, is what we should do.

That is what positive pressure can do.

There are many ways you can use pressure as a powerful motivating force to achieve your goals. For example, I recently talked to a friend who told me he made an appointment with a photographer for 12 weeks from the day he started his Program. He paid the photographer in advance and, to create a penalty for not meeting his deadline, signed a letter stating if he didn't show up for his photo shoot on that date, the photographer could keep the money. That penalty created pressure, which became a very real part of his incentive.

I've heard from other people who have harnessed the power of positive pressure by simply telling friends, family members, and co-workers about the deadlines for their goals. These people discovered that this extra push kept them from giving up because they didn't want to be seen as quitters—they wanted to honor their word to themselves and to others.

Another way to utilize the power of positive pressure is to enter some type of competition. Competition is a powerful force that can bring out the best in people, especially when there's something on the line. Look at any group of weekend warriors engaged in a trivial game of softball or one-on-one basketball. Having something at stake, like a trophy, turns up the pressure.

Unfortunately, most people who make a goal of building a better body don't set a deadline for achieving that objective, much less one that carries any type of reward or penalty. Therefore, the extraordinary motivating power of positive pressure is not harnessed.

odyforlife.com   www.bodyforlife.com   www.bodyforlife.com   www.bodyforlife.com   www.bodyforlife.com   www.bodyforlife.c

So, if at any point during the next 12 weeks, you pull back and start "coasting" and hoping success will just come to you, you're going to be extremely disappointed. In order to become our next real-life success story, you're going to need to harness the power of positive pressure. It's the antidote for breaking out of your comfort zone, which in reality is a very *uncomfortable* place to live.

──────── Focus on Progress, Not Perfection ────────

Now that you've begun your Program, it's vitally important that you protect your confidence. One way to do that is to forget about the whole concept of perfection. It doesn't exist. I've learned that chasing after perfection is as futile as trying to find the pot of gold at the end of a rainbow.

You see, perfection is an illusion, and if your objective is to achieve perfection in any aspect of this Program, you may end up with a sense of deficiency and uncertainty, which is *not* what you want.

If you don't strongly believe in what you're doing—if you cannot overcome feelings of self-doubt—it doesn't matter how much accurate information about training and nutrition you have. Without confidence, you won't be able to stay on course.

Think of the athlete who's having a great game until he makes a mistake. He throws an interception that is returned by the opposing team for a touchdown; he misses a critical free throw; he strikes out in a key situation. In a matter of seconds, he can plummet from extreme confidence to uncertainty and ineffectiveness.

If he doesn't know how to get his confidence back, he'll fall into a slump. He'll lose his energy. He'll stop playing to win, and instead, he will begin playing "not to lose."

Athletes aren't the only ones who need to maintain a strong sense of confidence in order to excel. Actors, artists, businessmen—all of us—we're at our

.bodyforlife.com   www.bodyforlife.com   www.bodyforlife.com   www.bodyforlife.com   www.bodyforlife.com   www.bodyforlif

best only when we're operating from a confident Power Mindset. Take virtually all successful people, extract their sense of certainty, and you'll strip them of everything else that has put them where they are—their talent, their drive, their energy, their judgment, their insight.

On the other hand, if you take people who are struggling—who are uncertain of themselves—and give them a healthy dose of confidence, their lives will turn inside out for the better, and fast. And that's what happens when you focus on *progress*. Even when you don't get everything "just right," you'll still feel strong. You'll still maintain your confidence and momentum.

One of the surefire ways to stay on track is to measure your progress often, which you can do literally every day with your Daily Progress Reports. I also recommend that you evaluate your success every four weeks by having your photo taken and your body composition measured. This will help you *maintain* your momentum and stay on course.

—— Practice the Universal Law of Reciprocation ——

To make the transformation in your life that you've now decided to make, sometime during these 12 weeks, you're going to need support. I believe the best way to receive it is to *give it*. That's called practicing the Universal Law of Reciprocation.

If you've never heard of this "law," you're not alone, even though it is the oldest rule in the book. It's at the center of virtually every religious, moral, and ethical system in the world. But it's missing from many of our lives, and this lack can keep us from fulfilling our potential.

Many people want to get before they give. In the long run, this formula never works. My experience has been this: When I focus on creating value for others, in either my personal or my professional life, I don't get back a return that merely equals what I invest. I know my return will be double, triple, even 10 times greater. This is such a fundamental truth that I don't even think about

bodyforlife.com   www.bodyforlife.com   www.bodyforlife.com   www.bodyforlife.com   www.bodyforlife.com   www.bodyforlife.c

it. I don't pay attention to my future return. The payoff will be automatic. And it will come in many forms: satisfaction, pride, fun, fulfillment, friendship, self-esteem, energy. And sometimes, yes, money.

There are many ways in which you can put the Universal Law of Reciprocation to work for you. First make a self-promise to do something positive for two people whom you would like to support you in your effort to make the next 12 weeks a success.

For example, you might think about one of the special things your husband or wife, or your mother or father, or your children do to add value to your life. (Don't focus on the little things they might do that aren't "perfect." See only what's right for a moment.)

Then, promise yourself you will share this positive thought with that person by the end of the day tomorrow. You can do this in person or by simply writing a brief note on a card or a piece of paper (written, appreciative words have enormous power) and sending it to them.

This simple exercise creates immediate results that will increase your energy and confidence and show you what a difference it makes when you look for what's right in someone instead of what's wrong. When you say something as simple as, "I appreciate your support," you not only lift that person's spirit but, as dictated by the Universal Law of Reciprocation, you will receive more positive energy than you give. That's the way it always has and always will work.

Begin the process of being a purveyor of positive energy with your family and friends, but don't stop there. You can practice this same exercise whenever and wherever you want, to create a more positive environment wherever you are. If you're feeling a little uncertain at work, or in the gym, look for something good in two people you come in contact with and make a point of saying something sincere and supportive.

Say you see someone at the gym who you can tell is making a great effort to improve him or herself. By simply telling him, "It looks like you're making some excellent progress. I admire your hard work," you will not only lift that person's energy, but you'll feel more confident as well.

bodyforlife.com   www.bodyforlife.com   www.bodyforlife.com   www.bodyforlife.com   www.bodyforlife.com   www.bodyforlife

You can also build energy and confidence by giving to a worthwhile cause, which, as you may or may not know, you have already started. You see, any proceeds that would have gone to me from the sale of this book are going instead to a charity I strongly believe in, the Make-A-Wish Foundation® of Colorado. Their mission is to create special memories and moments of happiness in the lives of children and their families around the world—lives that have been shattered by cancer, muscular dystrophy, heart disease, and other serious illnesses. These kids' days are filled with doctors, hospitals, medical treatments, and prognoses far removed from the wonder of normal childhood.

I could go on and on about how much I admire the courage of the Make-A-Wish children and all the unselfish people who support this cause, including each and every one of the thousands of readers of my magazine who have donated to my *Body of Work* fund-raiser for the Make-A-Wish Foundation®, which has already brought in over $1.25 million. Thanks to their generosity, the Make-A-Wish Foundation® has been able to grant more than 50,000 wishes.

What cause you support is entirely up to you. It could be a charity, a church, or an individual who needs your help. There is no shortage of worthwhile causes to get involved in. I know you will find one you can feel passionate about. And remember, you don't have to donate money to support a cause; you can volunteer your time, your talent, or resources you have access to that might help out. The important thing is to give often and not expect anything in return.

I know from my own experiences that nothing is more rewarding than to know you have made a difference in someone else's life. And I believe that when you finish this Body-*for*-LIFE Program, you will inspire others to follow in your footsteps. People will recognize you as a leader, and you will earn a new level of admiration and respect from your family, your friends, and others. Your success will help fuel their desire and give them hope that they too have the power to change.

The bottom line is this: You do have the power to inspire others, and in return, they will inspire you—they will help support you.

.bodyforlife.com   www.bodyforlife.com   www.bodyforlife.com   www.bodyforlife.com   www.bodyforlife.com   www.bodyforlife

We're Here for *You*

Remember at the beginning of this book when I promised you that if you let me, I would do anything and everything I could to help you transform your Body-*for*-LIFE? Well, I *really* meant that. And yet another one of the ways I can help you is by providing access to our Body-*for*-LIFE Line™—it's a *free* service we provide where you can call, 24 hours a day, 7 days a week, 365 days a year, and talk to people who have successfully completed a 12-week Body-*for*-LIFE Program—who have already walked a mile in your shoes, so to speak. The number is 1-800-297-9776 (Dept. #11).

Our Support Team is available to answer questions you have—whether they pertain to Crossing the Abyss, the Training-*for*-LIFE Experience, or the Eating-*for*-LIFE Method.

Also, you can call our Body-*for*-LIFE Line and share your progress on a daily, weekly, or monthly basis. (One of the most *heartbreaking* things for me is to see someone who is making extraordinary progress on this Program but who has no one to celebrate with.) We'd *love* to hear about your success and help celebrate *your* progress.

Also, you can visit our website at www.bodyforlife.com (the "com" stands for *community*) to receive daily advice and share your success with others who are following the Body-*for*-LIFE Program. You can also review new success stories every day, as well as review my answers to questions about the Program.

And most important of all, if you *ever* think of quitting, if, for any reason, you feel you can't continue the journey you've started, *please* contact us and let us help you. *Don't give up on yourself. Please* don't quit. Remember, you are *not* alone. We are here to *help you succeed.*

v.bodyforlife.com   www.bodyforlife.com   www.bodyforlife.com   www.bodyforlife.com   **www.bodyforlife.com**   www.bodyforlife

Overview of Staying on Course

- Expect adversity and be prepared to transform obstacles into energy.

- Honor self-promises by finishing what you start.

- Harness the power of positive pressure by embracing challenges.

- Focus on progress, not perfection in order to build confidence.

- Practice the Universal Law of Reciprocation by giving unselfishly.

- Let our Body-*for*-LIFE Support Team help you succeed.

bodyforlife.com   www.bodyforlife.com   www.bodyforlife.com   www.bodyforlife.com   www.bodyforlife.com   www.bodyforlife.

The Gateway

The Dream: Change the world . . . one life at a time.
The Goal: Transform one million Bodies-for-LIFE by 12/31/01.

So now we're finished, right?

No way.

I've said it from the beginning, and now *you* know it as well (you've *got* to, if you've read all these pages, if you've *really* read them): The 12-week journey you're about to begin with your body is merely a *gateway* to the rest of your life, a life of rewarding and fulfilling moments, perhaps more spectacular than you've ever dared to dream before.

You are in the process now—and yes, it's *already* begun—of *proving* to yourself that astounding changes *are* within your grasp. Within 12 weeks, you are going to know—not *believe*, but *know*—that the transformation you've created with your body is merely an example of the power you have to transform *everything else in your world*.

And here's the kicker:

You are not alone.

There is something afoot in our society, a gathering force that is beginning to rise as the twenty-first century begins. People are reaching as they have

111

never reached before. They are searching. They are hungry for hope, for meaning, for clarity, for something to believe in. And they are discovering that search, that *belief*, has got to begin with *themselves*.

That's what this book is about.

People have had enough of fragmentation, of coming apart—both as individuals and as communities. They have had enough of conflict—of fighting one another and of fighting *themselves*. We have seen what happens when we separate ourselves from one another and when we separate ourselves from our *selves*. We have seen the decay that takes place when we neglect our bodies, and now we know that it is a metaphor for the decay that takes place in any and every aspect of our lives that goes without care or attention.

The process of picking up the broken pieces of our selves and our society has begun. But, we are not merely putting them back together: We are now *re-creating* them, making them stronger and better than before.

That is what our society—and I dare say the world—is doing as this millennium draws to a close. We are transforming. We are beginning to celebrate our progress, our lives, each and every day. We are looking to the future with optimism, a sense of confidence, of potential, of promise . . . *of beginning*.

As we cross over into the new millennium, people everywhere are feeling it. They're living it. Make no mistake, it *is* happening. It's happening in families, in neighborhoods, in schools, in churches, at the workplace—in each and every community.

People are discovering that they *do* have the power to change. That they *do* have the ability to create not only a better body but a better *life*, for themselves *and* others. They are no longer saying, "It's beyond me; it's out of my control." They've stopped asking or expecting *someone else* to do what needs to be done for them.

They are beginning to do it for themselves.

And, they are helping one another.

bodyforlife.com   www.bodyforlife.com   www.bodyforlife.com   www.bodyforlife.com   www.bodyforlife.com   www.bodyforlife.

If there are two fundamental messages that lie at the foundation of this book and this Program—and indeed of *my life* and, I hope, *yours*—it is these two principles:

- The more you create value for others—the more you *reach out* and *give* to make their lives better—the *stronger* and *richer*, in every sense of those two words, your own life will become.

- *You* can regain control of *your* life and change it, *beginning with your body*, but only beginning there, and it will *all* begin to come your way as soon as you *decide* to let it.

These two principles are guiding the revolution—the *evolution* that *is* taking place. If you don't sense it at this moment, when you wake up 12 weeks from now and look in the mirror, will you say, "I wish I had…" or "I'm glad I did…"?

But I believe you *do* sense it right now. You wouldn't be reading these words if you didn't. You have made the decision to become part of this change for the better, and for that, I both thank you and welcome you.

The success stories you've read in these pages—of changed bodies and lives—of ordinary people who've become extraordinary in ways they couldn't have imagined—are just the base of a mountain—a mountain of real-life transformations that reaches a higher point every day.

I've read thousands of letters, cards, faxes, and e-mails from these men and women. I meet them everywhere I go. They are *my* teachers, each and every one of them. They've lifted me higher than I ever dreamed I could rise. And they've inspired me to reach even higher—to achieve my goal of helping one million people transform their bodies and lives by December 31, 2001.

This is *my* goal—to help you achieve *your* goal.

I will do everything I can to educate and empower you not just to "get in shape" but to help you reach *higher* than you've ever dreamed you could reach—to achieve clarity, control, and confidence; to help you build and nurture your absolute best, your one and only *Body-for-LIFE!*

.bodyforlife.com www.bodyforlife.com www.bodyforlife.com www.bodyforlife.com www.bodyforlife.com www.bodyforlife

By working together, as a *team*, we can succeed, and *we will succeed.*

And now, finally, there is but one last promise I'd like you to make as we embark upon this 12-week transformation process. I'd like you to promise me—and yourself—that you'll contact me when you're finished and tell me what's begun.

Again, I welcome you, and I thank you.

bodyforlife.com   www.bodyforlife.com   www.bodyforlife.com   www.bodyforlife.com   www.bodyforlife.com   www.bodyforlife

Questions and Answers

Q: My 32-year-old daughter is about 30 pounds overweight. She's tried everything to get in shape—prescription diet pills, thigh creams, even liposuction. How can I help her?

A: What your daughter is doing is a common mistake. I call it "the outside-in approach." That's where you try to solve a problem by treating the symptoms, not the cause. It doesn't work.

The Liposuction has got to be the ultimate outside-in approach. I've thought about it quite a bit, and I can't think of any way that having a steel rod jammed under your skin and having fat sucked out of your body could possibly enhance your self-esteem.

The Body-*for*-LIFE Program is different because it takes an "*inside-out* approach." We start with the *inside*—your *reasons* for wanting to change: your dreams, your goals, your life. A successful transformation always starts on the inside.

Q: I can't find time to exercise, but I need to lose 25 pounds of fat. What should I do?

A: Here's a secret—I can't *find* time to exercise either. Neither can John Elway. Neither can Sylvester Stallone. Neither can David Kennedy, a friend of

w.bodyforlife.com   www.bodyforlife.com   www.bodyforlife.com   www.bodyforlife.com   **www.bodyforlife.com**   www.bodyforlif

mine who's a sergeant in the Army. Neither can Russell Simpson, who's a father and a medical doctor. Neither can Christy Hammons, who's a college student and works at night to earn money to pay her tuition.

In fact, out of the 611,000 people who have come to me over the last two years and asked for my help, not a single one of them has said anything remotely like, "Bill, I don't have much to do with my days . . . I figured I'd start exercising . . . can you help me kill some time?"

The inverse is always true—in this fast-paced, dynamic, hectic, rapidly changing world in which we all live, virtually no one thinks he or she can find time for anything new. But that's a *misperception*. And let me warn you that whatever you *perceive*, you *believe*. You see, as much as we might try to convince ourselves that we are simply too busy, that's just not the case. Believe it or not, people who are remarkably successful at transforming their bodies and lives have exactly 24 hours in every day, just like you and I do. There's not a single person on the planet who's figured out how to get more out of a day than 1,440 minutes.

So why do some people seem to have more space in those 24 hours than others? Remember what I taught you about *transforming* patterns of action back on page 29? Well, that's what we're doing here—we're looking for habits that might be taking up time that is not taking us closer to achieving our goals, and we're transforming those patterns. For example, if you can take just four hours a week that you spend watching TV and use that time, instead, for exercise, you've created a solution to this perceived problem.

Another thing you can do to create time is schedule your workouts and plan everything you're going to do each day. You see, if you have no idea what you're going to do tomorrow, until tomorrow comes, you'll wind up wasting a lot of time reacting, adjusting, and trying to figure out just exactly what to do, when to do it, or how to do it. When you plan ahead, you eliminate a lot of unnecessary problems.

Now, of course, you can't plan everything. But scheduling your time takes only a few minutes a night, and you can easily pick up an hour you

odyforlife.com　www.bodyforlife.com　www.bodyforlife.com　www.bodyforlife.com　www.bodyforlife.com　www.bodyforlife.c

didn't know you had. Another thing you can do to create more time is exercise. Yes, *exercise*. It's a scientific fact that the proper amount of exercise creates energy. When you have more energy, you get more done, faster.

Q: How do I keep up with my workouts while I'm traveling?

A: Before you travel, you must *plan*. Find out if the hotel you're staying in has an exercise facility or at least a set of dumbbells. If not, find out where the closest gym is to where you're staying, and *plan* when you'll work out.

You'll find a decent gym in virtually every city in America, and most hotels have a "fitness area" of some kind or at least a set of dumbbells.

Also, decide beforehand to overcome whatever adversity you face. If living a healthy, fulfilling life is a priority to you, you will succeed.

Q: What do I do after 12 weeks?

A: Once you've completed this 12-week journey, it's highly unlikely that you will even *imagine* reverting to your old ways. You will *literally* be a changed person. What feels "normal" to you will be different: your dreams, your passions, your cravings, your pleasures. They will all be redefined. And they will be rooted in the *new* you—your new patterns, your new lifestyle, your new outlook, energy and optimism, and yes, your new *body*.

Imagine if you learned you had been walking incorrectly all your life, and *that* was why you felt pain and distress in your legs and back at the end of every day and why you woke up weary and sore each morning. Imagine that you were then shown how to walk correctly, and the pain and fatigue disappeared. Why in the world would you *ever* choose to go back to walking the way you used to? Well, that's precisely the way people feel after they've gone through this Program. For them, it becomes a way of life.

With that in mind, what I recommend is, after 12 weeks, set new goals for the next 12 weeks and continue to look and move forward. What I think you'll find is the first 12 weeks are the most challenging because, for many,

v.bodyforlife.com   www.bodyforlife.com   www.bodyforlife.com   www.bodyforlife.com   www.bodyforlife.com   www.bodyforlife

it requires breaking numerous patterns and climbing a pretty steep learning curve. Comparatively, your second 12 weeks will be a breeze, your third will be a way of *life*.

Q: What if I make a mistake and miss a workout or meal?

A: If you miss a workout, you missed it. If you miss a meal, you missed it. Just get back on schedule and keep moving forward. And *please* do not let setbacks or "mistakes" slow you down. We've *all* made mistakes in the past, and we're all going to make mistakes in the future, especially if we're trying something new and challenging. So, let's start making 'em. Because if we're making mistakes, it means we're trying, and we're learning.

Q: I showed my trainer some of the before-and-after photos of people who followed your Program. He told me it takes at least *two years* to make a physique transformation like that. Is he right?

A: You know that saying, "I'll believe it when I see it"? Well, like most maxims, it has exceptions. What I've observed is that some people can only see it *after* they believe it.

You see, one of the first steps to making a change is to *believe* it can be done. And I'm not just talking about getting psyched up for a few minutes, a few hours, or even a few days. I'm talking about *truly believing*.

The truth is, tens of thousands of people have already dramatically transformed their physiques in as little as 12 weeks, and tens of thousands more are doing it right now—burning more fat and building more strength in a matter of months than they have in years.

So why do some grown men and women reject the truth?

Well, when you really get down to it, the person who disbelieves something that there's enormous social proof to support is not just experiencing healthy skepticism. It's actually a symptom of cynicism—that doubting mindset that robs people of the potential to transform or to accept that they too have the power to change.

bodyforlife.com   www.bodyforlife.com   www.bodyforlife.com   www.bodyforlife.com   www.bodyforlife.com   www.bodyforlife.

And the solution? For starters, you must open your mind. And you have to start setting and achieving goals. That will fuel your desire and let you dream—to be inspired.

The bottom line is, if *you* believe you can do it, then *you can*. And when you succeed, you'll inspire your trainer to believe it's possible; then he'll see it, too. (Pretty nifty how that works, huh?)

Q: How much fat should I expect to lose if I follow the Program for 12 weeks?

A: I've been tracking and researching this for years, and I believe most people can lose up to 25 pounds of body fat in 12 weeks, if that's the goal. If you're losing more weight than two pounds a week, you may be losing muscle tissue as well, which is bad news—remember, if you lose muscle, your metabolism will slow down, and your fat loss could come to a screeching halt.

Although it's rare for someone to lose more than 25 pounds of body weight (notice I didn't say body fat) in 12 weeks, without losing muscle, it's not impossible: Some people's bodies are so far out of whack—they're holding so much water—that once they start the Program, their bodies just completely readjust.

Don't forget what we're trying to accomplish is a reduction in body *fat*, not just body weight—there's a big difference. Your body weight is made up of lean body mass (muscle tissue, water, bone, internal organs), and your body fat is . . . well, it's *fat*.

Some fitness centers and hospitals now offer various methods of body-fat testing, but I think the most convenient way to do it is to use something called "skin-fold calipers." You simply pinch your skin at certain sites with this device, and it helps you calculate the amount of body fat you have.

You can buy a set of skin-fold calipers called the Accu-Measure, which cost only about $20 by calling a company called Body Trends Health and Fitness at 1-800-549-1667, or visit their website at www.bodytrends.com.

v.bodyforlife.com   www.bodyforlife.com   www.bodyforlife.com   www.bodyforlife.com   www.bodyforlife.com   www.bodyforlif

Or you can buy a set of Slim Guide skin-fold calipers for around $20 by calling a company called Fitnessesities at 1-800-942-8436, or visit their website at www.fitnessesities.com.

Be sure to measure your body fat every four weeks and have your photo taken (in a pair of shorts or a bathing suit). This will help you chart your progress.

Q: Can I listen to music while I work out? If so, what kind is best?

A: Of course you can listen to music while you work out—the "best" kind is whatever you like: Rock, jazz, opera. It's up to you. Sometimes I listen to music; sometimes I listen to books on tape while I work out. Sometimes I like it quiet.

Q: I'm naturally very lean. I don't need to lose fat. Can I use the Body-*for*-LIFE Program to gain muscle size and strength?

A: The Body-*for*-LIFE Program described in this book is designed to help you build your best body *and* enhance your mental and physical strength. It's really about so much more than building muscle—it's about building a stronger *life*.

That being said, for those who are naturally very lean and whose goals include gaining muscle size and strength but not losing fat, I suggest you follow the Training-*for*-LIFE Experience and the Eating-*for*-LIFE Method, and for your first three meals of the day, include two carbohydrate portions instead of one. This extra energy intake will ensure that the fuel required to build muscle is available when and where it's needed because if you are *very* lean (below seven percent body fat for men and below 12 percent body fat for women), the energy required to build muscle may not be pulled from stored body fat; therefore, it must be provided through your food intake.

For example, instead of having an egg-white omelet (a portion of protein) and a grapefruit (a portion of carbohydrate) for breakfast, you would have that *plus* a bowl of oatmeal (a second portion of carbohydrates). And, for your mid-morning meal, instead of having a Myoplex

odyforlife.com   www.bodyforlife.com   www.bodyforlife.com   www.bodyforlife.com   www.bodyforlife.com   www.bodyforlife.c

Performance-Nutrition Shake (which contains a portion of protein and carbohydrates), you would have that plus a portion of yogurt. And, for lunch, instead of having a grilled chicken breast (a portion of protein), a baked potato (a portion of carbohydrates), and steamed spinach (a vegetable portion [remember, you should have a vegetable portion with at least two of your six daily meals]), you can have that, plus a serving of pasta.

Another thing that could help you gain muscle size and strength faster is to use an EAS supplement called Phosphagen HP, which is very popular among athletes who are trying to gain muscle size and strength. This supplement contains creatine, a nutrient which has been shown, in dozens of university studies, to enhance size and muscle strength, as well as energy. University studies have shown that Phosphagen HP (a unique blend of creatine plus energy-rich carbohydrates and other nutrients that enhance the transport of creatine to muscle cells) may work even better than plain creatine.

The other supplement I recommend to enhance the muscle-building effects of the Training-*for*-LIFE Experience is called HMB (beta-hydroxy beta-methylbutyrate). This is a nutrient which university studies have shown enhances the positive effects of intense exercise, and, like creatine, it is extremely popular with athletes.

The only supplements I'm using right now are Myoplex Performance-Nutrition Shakes and an EAS supplement called BetaGen (which contains *both* creatine and HMB). BetaGen is a powdered drink mix that I usually just add to Myoplex. When I consume these supplements, I get the vitamins, minerals, protein, extra antioxidants, creatine, HMB, glutamine (an important amino acid that helps with muscle metabolism), energy-rich carbohydrates, and other micronutrients I need. I don't make it any more complicated than that.

Now remember, supplements alone will not help you build a better body. You have to cross the abyss and *apply* your knowledge of exercise and nutrition.

.bodyforlife.com   www.bodyforlife.com   www.bodyforlife.com   www.bodyforlife.com   **www.bodyforlife.com**   www.bodyforlife

By the way, for those of you who are interested in the science of performance nutrition and supplementation, you can find detailed scientific information, including dozens of peer-reviewed studies and research reports at www.eas.com.

Q: Is the 20-Minute Aerobics Solution really enough to burn fat?

A: Yes. Remember, it's not just the amount of calories you burn during the exercises session, it's the amount you burn the hour after as well.

Q: Is it true once you have cellulite on your thighs, you can never get rid of it?

A: Although some "experts" insist cellulite is a "medical syndrome" you're stuck with, I disagree. And I know several thousand women who will back me up—women who have successfully completed this Program and lost cellulite. The fact is, when you lose fat, you lose cellulite. And when you follow this Program, you'll lose fat, and you'll build *firm* muscle.

Q: The last thing I feel like doing in the morning is exercising. Can't I do my aerobics at night?

A: The temptation to eat muffins and drink coffee may be overwhelming (just as going back to bed might be) first thing in the morning, but keep this in mind: Doing intense aerobic exercise on an empty stomach for just 20 minutes first thing in the morning is more effective in burning fat than *a full hour* of aerobic exercise performed later in the day after you've eaten a few meals. You see, after an overnight fast, blood-sugar levels are low, as are carbohydrate reserves. Exercising before you eat causes the body to dip right into stored fat to come up with the energy required to make it through whatever rude awakening you've subjected it to.

Now, if you just can't do your aerobic exercise in the morning, the next best thing is to do it in the evening, after not eating for three hours. For example, if you plan to conduct the 20-Minute Aerobic Solution at 6:30 P.M., have a protein- and carbohydrate-containing meal at 3:30 P.M. Then eat again an hour after your workout.

bodyforlife.com   www.bodyforlife.com   www.bodyforlife.com   www.bodyforlife.com   www.bodyforlife.com   www.bodyforlife.

Q: Can I exercise at home and still follow the Body-*for*-LIFE Program? If so, what kind of equipment do I need?

A: You can put together an excellent home gym with a quality set of dumbbells and an exercise bench you can buy at any sporting goods store. What you'll probably need is a set of adjustable dumbbells that go as light as 2.5 pounds and up to 30, 40, or 50 pounds each (depending on your level of strength, of course). You'll also need to invest in an adjustable exercise bench. Compared with most home-exercise equipment, dumbbells and a bench are a bargain. Take a look at just some of the advantages of using dumbbells:

• Dumbbells permit individualized and optimized alignment of joints, making the exercises both safer and more effective. In other words, the dumbbells fit you; you don't have to fit yourself to a machine or its movement.

• Dumbbells allow wrists and elbows to be in the most natural position and to rotate throughout the range of motion of exercises involving your upper body.

• Dumbbells allow upper body exercises, like presses, to occur in arcs, which are the most natural way for our bodies to move—thus increasing the range of motion of all exercises, which potentially allows for greater improvements in flexibility, while enhancing coordination and balance.

• Dumbbells permit the greatest possible variety of exercises. Most can be learned quickly and performed easily by men and women of all fitness levels.

• Dumbbells work the muscles which help stabilize the joints along with the primary movers for each exercise, contributing to total body development.

• Dumbbells permit a faster workout, contributing to workout efficiency, calorie burning, and overall aerobic and cardiovascular benefits of the workout.

• Dumbbell training is inherently safe. I've never observed a torn muscle or any other serious injury resulting from the proper use of dumbbells.

.bodyforlife.com   www.bodyforlife.com   www.bodyforlife.com   www.bodyforlife.com   www.bodyforlife.com   www.bodyforlife

Q: I have trouble finding time during the week to prepare healthy meals. How can I stick with this?

A: Most of us are too busy to prepare healthy, low-fat foods every day: That's the secret to the success of fast-food restaurants. One possible solution would be to prepare some low-fat protein- and carbohydrate-balanced meals on Sunday night or whenever you have some extra time and then freeze them. Then, just take them out and put them in the microwave for a few minutes whenever you need them, and you're all set.

Another way to make it a lot easier to consume six meals a day is to consume three regular, whole-food meals, each consisting of a portion of protein and carbohydrates, and protein-rich, low-fat nutrition shakes or bars for the other three meals.

Remember, by feeding your body frequently throughout the day, you can avoid hunger cramps and maintain stable energy levels and a healthy metabolism. It's also a great way to provide your body with the nutrients it needs to recover from weight-training exercise and squelch cravings, especially those uncontrollable urges to binge during the evening.

Q: Is it all right to drink wine with my evening meals?

A: An occasional glass or two of wine is fine. But you must use moderation. Beer and wine drinkers are often reluctant to give up the beverage of their choice. Case in point: Last summer I was trying to help a guy who couldn't lose fat "no matter what." I discovered he was eating right, but he was also drinking a six-pack of beer each night. Do that every night, and you'll put on six to 10 pounds of unhealthy fat a month.

Q: My unfit friends always try to get me to eat unhealthy foods when we go out. It's hard to say no. What should I do?

A: Don't fall prey to the same eating habits that may have had something to do with making your friends unfit in the first place. If you eat with people with poor eating habits, you must be careful not to use their

bodyforlife.com   www.bodyforlife.com   www.bodyforlife.com   www.bodyforlife.com   www.bodyforlife.com   www.bodyforlife

dietary shortcomings to justify slipping into similar eating patterns. Turn the tables, so to speak—influence them to improve their eating habits by explaining your reasons for making a change and let them know you'll support them if they're interested in improving the way they look and feel.

Or try to visit with those friends on your free day—that one day a week when you can eat whatever you like—apple pie, French fries, pizza, etc.

Q: Is it okay to eat frozen yogurt?

A: Do not mistake frozen yogurt for a health food. Not all frozen yogurt is low fat. Some varieties average about eight grams of fat per cup. Secondly, there's hardly any way of telling what the fat content is of the local neighborhood yogurt stand's frozen offerings. Therefore, I recommend you eat frozen yogurt only on your free days.

Q: Should I eat something before I work out, like an energy bar?

A: It depends on what your goal is. If your only concern is athletic performance, you should consume carbohydrates like energy bars and/or sports drinks, before, during, and after you engage in physical activity.

However, if your goal is to lose fat and gain muscle, I do not recommend eating before you work out. This is a mistake a lot of people make. If you supply the body with carbohydrates to use as fuel when exercising, it will prevent fat burning and preserve body-fat stores. A recent study confirmed that if you keep taking in carbs, your body will burn carbs. Cut back on the carbs, and your body will burn fat more readily and quickly. That's why I recommend, for maximum fat-burning effect, you exercise on an empty stomach.

Q: Should my teenage boys start this Program?

A: The Body-*for*-LIFE Program is intended for healthy adults—generally those over the age of 18.

I do not believe young teens—ages 13 to 15—should train with weights. At that age, I recommend calisthenics, like jumping jacks, push-ups, pull-ups, sit-ups, and running—the type of activity I used to do when I was that age.

.bodyforlife.com   www.bodyforlife.com   www.bodyforlife.com   www.bodyforlife.com   www.bodyforlife.com   www.bodyforlife

Sixteen- and 17-year-olds can do the exercises described in this book, but their aim should be to conduct 15 to 25 repetitions per set, and using the Intensity Index (page 62), they should never exceed a level 7 effort. You see, during puberty, the body is so primed for growth that low-intensity resistance exercise creates results. But, during puberty, the bones are still growing, and strenuous resistance exercise may interfere with bone growth; thus, teenagers should *not* begin working out *intensely* with weights until they have completely "matured" physically. Typically that's around age 18.

In terms of nutrition, I believe teenagers should develop the habit of eating frequent, high-nutrient, protein- and carbohydrate-containing meals. However, fast-growing teenagers should not restrict calories—as long as the food is of good quality (chicken, potatoes, rice, fruit, vegetables, milk), they should eat often and plentifully.

As for teens and supplements, when something's working right, why mess with it? So when kids ask me about whether they should use creatine or whatever, I say forget it. Invest in a good healthy diet. Eat the right foods six times a day. Avoid the wrong foods. And drink a lot of water.

Q: Can I still eat cheese with this nutrition method?

A: Cheese is usually too high in fat, so I don't recommend it, but if you're preparing a "healthy" dish that requires it, try defatting your cheese—zap an ounce of full-fat cheddar in the microwave on the high setting for two minutes, and much of the fat will liquefy and form a pool on top of the cheese. You can then pour the fat off. This method will get rid of more than half the fat in cheese. (It works best with cheddar or mozzarella.)

Q: The gym I belong to has over 100 exercise machines which look very high-tech. Do these work?

A: Please do not be distracted by all those fancy exercise machines. Which ones work? Which don't? *Who knows?* It's guesswork—trial and error. All you need from a gym to follow the Training-*for*-LIFE Experience are barbells, dumbbells, benches, and a few *standard* machines, like a high-cable

bodyforlife.com   www.bodyforlife.com   www.bodyforlife.com   www.bodyforlife.com   www.bodyforlife.com   www.bodyforlife.

pulley, leg extension, leg curl, leg press, and squat rack. The basic free-weight exercises shown in the Exercise Guide on page 136 work for me, and they *will* work for you too. In fact, the vast majority of elite athletes I work with stick with the *basics* as well.

Q: I've read the success stories from people who have competed in your challenges, and I'd like to take part. Can I enter?

A: My annual Transformation Challenges are for people from all walks of life—young and old, fit and unfit, men and women. The rules are simple: Follow the Body-*for*-LIFE Program for 12 weeks and document your results with before-and-after photos and body-composition tests.

Then, write an essay about how this experience has affected your body and life. Your overall score will be based 50 percent on your body transformation and 50 percent on your essay. The competitors with the highest combined scores from our 10 judges win. That's all there is to it.

Our prize purse for 1999 includes $1 million in cash and 100 first-class, all-expenses-paid dream vacations to Hawaii. So if you're looking for an extra incentive to put the Body-*for*-LIFE Program to the test, accepting my challenge may help. For details, call 1-800-297-9776 (Dept. #18) or visit www.bodyforlife.com to request your Rules & Regulations Kit, which will tell you everything you need to know about how to enter and win.

Q: I've tried to stick with an exercise program, but I've never been able to be consistent. I guess I just don't believe in exercise. Aren't some people just not cut out for it?

A: A lot of people tell me they just can't bring themselves to exercise regularly. "It's just too hard," they complain. "It's not for me." That's just not true. In fact, having the ability to move and *not* moving is just plain wrong.

Consider this . . .

I recently spent some time with a great young guy from Scottsdale, Arizona. His name is Jamie Brunner, and he's one of our newest

.bodyforlife.com   www.bodyforlife.com   www.bodyforlife.com   www.bodyforlife.com   www.bodyforlife.com   www.bodyforlife.

Transformation Challenge Champions. Jamie's 25 years old. He's married to a beautiful, young woman. And he's smart. But he had allowed himself to balloon up to 235 pounds—to get, in other words, "downright fat." (Those are his words, not mine.)

Anyway, Jamie has an older brother named Barry whom he looks up to. Growing up, they always hung out together. They're best friends.

One day, a few years back, Jamie and Barry went swimming in a lake. Barry dove in the water, not knowing there was a rock just below the surface. He broke his neck—shattered what they call the C2 and C3 vertebrae. Ever since, he's been paralyzed from the neck down. It was a tragic accident that, as you might imagine, has taken a lot of healing to cope with.

Jamie explained to me that one day he was talking with Barry about the difficulty he was experiencing trying to get in shape. He told his brother, "I can't stand running on the treadmill or lifting weights. I just hate it!" To which Barry responded, "Jamie, I'd give anything in the *world* to run on a treadmill. I'd give anything in the world to flex the muscles in my legs—to feel my arms getting stronger—to feel them *move*. I'd give anything to have the *choice* that you have—to move, to lift, to run . . . but I *don't* have that choice. If you won't do it for yourself, Jamie, do it for me."

Jamie was speechless. He told me he never felt so selfish in his life. How could he complain to his brother, who can't even raise his hand, that exercising is an inconvenience, that moving the body is a "pain"? Jamie told me that was the turning point for him, and he has never missed a workout since.

Jamie's breakthrough made me think, too. I realized that having a healthy body and letting it decay, having the *ability* to exercise and *not* doing it, is like having 20/20 vision and never opening your eyes. Fortunately, more and more people are beginning to see it that way.

Terms and Jargon

Abyss: A barrier which stands between knowing what needs to be done and actually doing it.

Aerobic: This means "requiring oxygen." Aerobic metabolism occurs during low-intensity, long-duration exercises, like jogging.

Amino acids: A group of compounds that serve as the building blocks from which protein and muscle are made.

Anaerobic: This means "without oxygen." Anaerobic metabolism in muscle tissue occurs during intense physical activities like sprinting or weight lifting.

Antioxidants: Small compounds that minimize tissue oxidation and help control free radicals and their negative effects.

Atrophy: A decrease in size or "wasting away" of muscle tissue from lack of use.

Barbell: A free weight consisting of a long bar on which weight plates are placed. It is normally lifted with both arms.

Body composition: The percentage of your body weight composed of fat compared to fat-free mass.

Calories: The unit for measuring the energy value of foods.

129

Carbohydrates: Organic compounds containing carbon, hydrogen, and oxygen. They're a very effective fuel source for the body. The different types of carbohydrates include starches, sugars, and fibers. Carbohydrates contain four calories per gram. Glucose—blood sugar—is a carbohydrate used by every cell in the body as fuel.

Cholesterol: A type of fat that, although most widely known as a "bad fat" implicated in promoting heart disease and stroke, is a vital component in the production of many hormones in the body. There are different types of cholesterol: namely, HDL and LDL (HDL being the "good" form and LDL being the "bad" form).

Clean diet: This refers to eating nutrient-rich, low-fat meals.

Concentric: The lifting phase of an exercise, when the muscle shortens or contracts. For example, when you lift the weight in a bench press, pressing it from your chest to the lock-out position, that's the concentric, or "positive," phase of the exercise.

Deficiency: A suboptimal level of one or more nutrients that are essential for good health, most often seen with vitamins. A deficiency can be caused by poor nutrition, increased bodily demands (especially from intense training), or both.

Diet: Food and drink regularly consumed by a person, often according to specific guidelines to improve physical condition.

Dumbbell: A free weight made up of a short handle on which weight plates are placed. These are normally lifted with one arm.

Eccentric: The lowering phase of an exercise, when the muscle lengthens. For example, lowering the weight to your chest during the bench press is the eccentric, or "negative," portion of the exercise.

Energy: The capacity to do work. Energy harnessed is power.

bodyforlife.com   www.bodyforlife.com   www.bodyforlife.com   www.bodyforlife.com   www.bodyforlife.com   www.bodyforlife

Essential fatty acids (EFAs): Fats our bodies can't make, so we must obtain them through our diets. These fats (which include linoleic and linolenic acid) are very important to hormone production, as well as cellular synthesis and integrity. Good sources of these fats are flaxseed oil and safflower oil.

Fat: One of the macronutrients. Fat contains nine calories per gram; it has the most calories of all the macronutrients. There are two types of fat—saturated "bad" fat and unsaturated "good" fat.

Fat-free mass (FFM): The part of the body not containing fat, including: bone, muscle, skin, organs, water, hair, blood, and lymph.

Free day: A day on the Body-*for*-LIFE Program when you must eat the foods you've craved the previous six days and must not exercise.

Frequent feeding: Eating often throughout the day to work with your body, not against it. By eating at regular intervals throughout the day (approximately every two to three hours), you can keep your metabolism elevated and energy levels stable.

Fructose: The main type of sugar found in fruit. It's sweeter than sucrose (table sugar).

Glucose: The simplest sugar molecule. It's also the main sugar found in blood and is used as a basic fuel for the body.

Glycogen: The principal stored form of carbohydrate energy (glucose), which is reserved in muscles. When your muscles are full of glycogen, they look and feel full.

Gorging: This refers to eating large amounts of food at one meal, then waiting for many hours, maybe a full day, before eating again. This is also known as bingeing.

Grazing: This term refers to frequent feedings—eating small amounts of food often.

w.bodyforlife.com   www.bodyforlife.com   www.bodyforlife.com   www.bodyforlife.com   www.bodyforlife.com   www.bodyforli

HDL: This stands for "high-density lipoprotein." It's one of the subcategories of cholesterol—typically thought of as the "good" cholesterol. You may be able to raise your HDL cholesterol levels by ingesting quality unsaturated fats like flaxseed oil. Exercise has also been shown to increase HDL levels.

Intensity: A measure of how much force or energy is put forth during a task.

Law of Nature: Use it or lose it.

Lean body mass (LBM): Another term which describes fat-free mass (see fat-free mass).

LDL: This stands for "low-density lipoprotein" and is a subcategory of cholesterol, typically thought of as the "bad" cholesterol. Levels of LDL cholesterol can be elevated by ingestion of saturated fats and a lack of exercise.

Linoleic acid: An essential fatty acid and, more specifically, an omega-6 polyunsaturated fatty acid. Good sources of this fatty acid are safflower oil and soybean oil.

Linolenic acid: An essential fatty acid and, more precisely, an omega-3 polyunsaturated fatty acid. It is found in high concentrations in flaxseed oil.

Meal: Food that's eaten at one time. Each meal should contain a portion (which is the size of the palm of your hand or your clenched fist) of protein and a portion of carbohydrates.

Metabolic rate: The rate you convert energy stores into working energy in your body. In other words, it's how fast your "whole system" runs. The metabolic rate is controlled by a number of factors, including: muscle mass (the greater your muscle mass, the greater your metabolic rate), calorie intake, and exercise.

Metabolism: The use of nutrients by the body. It's the process by which substances come into the body and the rate at which they are used.

odyforlife.com   www.bodyforlife.com   www.bodyforlife.com   www.bodyforlife.com   www.bodyforlife.com   www.bodyforlife.c

Minerals: Naturally occurring, inorganic substances that are essential for human life, which play a role in many vital metabolic processes.

Nutrients: Components of food that help nourish the body: that is, they provide energy or serve as "building materials." These nutrients include carbohydrates, fats, proteins, vitamins, minerals, water, etc.

Optimal nutrition: The best possible nutrition; distinct from merely adequate nutrition, which is characterized by no overt deficiency. This term describes people free from marginal deficiencies, imbalances, and toxicities, and who are not at risk for such.

Portion: The amount of carbohydrates or protein one should eat with each meal. A portion is the size of the palm of your hand or your clenched fist.

Power Mindset: The state of being where you feel self-reliant, confident, and strong.

Proteins: Proteins are the building blocks of muscle, enzymes, and some hormones. They are made up of amino acids and are essential for growth and repair in the body. A gram of protein contains four calories. Those from animal sources contain the essential amino acids. Those from vegetable sources contain some but not all of the essential amino acids. Proteins are broken up by the body to produce amino acids.

Repetition (rep): The number of times you lift and lower a weight in one set of an exercise. For example, if you lift and lower a weight 10 times before setting the weight down, you have completed 10 "reps" in one set.

Resistance exercise: Working out with weights or using your body to resist some other force. This includes a wide spectrum of motion, from push-ups to dumbbell curls.

Rest period: The amount of time you allow between sets and exercises.

Set: Group of reps (lifting and lowering a weight) of an exercise after which you take a brief rest period. For example, if you complete 10 reps, set the

.bodyforlife.com   www.bodyforlife.com   www.bodyforlife.com   www.bodyforlife.com   www.bodyforlife.com   www.bodyforlife

weight down, complete eight more reps, set the weight down again, and repeat for six more reps, you have completed three sets of the exercise.

Saturated fats: These are "bad" fats. They are called saturated because they contain no open spots on their carbon skeletons. These bad fats have been shown to raise cholesterol levels in the body. Sources of these fats include animal foods and hydrogenated vegetable oils, such as margarine.

Supplement: This is a term used to describe a preparation such as a tablet, pill, or powder that contains nutrients. Supplements are used to help you achieve optimal nutrient intake.

Unsaturated fats: These are "good" fats. They are called unsaturated because they have one or more open spots on their carbon skeletons. This category of fats includes the essential fatty acids linoleic and linolenic. The main sources of these fats are from plant foods, such as safflower, sunflower, and flaxseed oils.

Universal Law of Reciprocation: The more you help others, the more your life is enhanced.

Vitamins: Organic compounds that are vital to life, indispensable to bodily function, and needed in minute amounts. They are calorie-free essential nutrients. Many of them function as coenzymes, supporting a multitude of biological functions.

bodyforlife.com   www.bodyforlife.com   www.bodyforlife.com   www.bodyforlife.com   www.bodyforlife.com   www.bodyforlife.

Exercise Guide

Appendix C

Here's a list of 36 very effective weight-training exercises, which will work all the major muscle groups in your body (as shown on *my* body on the next page—of course, you have the same muscles in your body). On the pages that follow, you'll find complete, step-by-step instructions, which show how to do each of these result-producing exercises.

I realize this might seem somewhat overwhelming, but with a little practice, you *will* be able to properly conduct all of these exercises. Like learning how to ride a bike, once you know how to do it, you'll *always* know how to do it.

Chest	• dumbbell bench press • incline dumbbell press	• dumbbell flyes • barbell bench press
Shoulders	• seated dumbbell press • standing barbell press	• side raises • bent-over raises
Back	• wide-grip pulldowns • one-arm dumbbell rows	• reverse-grip pulldowns • dumbbell pullovers
Triceps	• dumbbell extensions • close-grip pushdowns	• bench dips • lying dumbbell extensions
Biceps	• incline dumbbell curls • seated dumbbell curls	• standing barbell curls • hammer curls
Quadriceps	• leg extensions • leg press	• barbell squats • dumbbell squats
Hamstrings	• dumbbell lunges • standing leg curls	• lying leg curls • straight-leg deadlifts
Calves	• seated calf raises • standing calf raises	• one-leg calf raises • angled calf raises
Abdominals	• floor crunches • twist crunches	• decline sit-ups • bent-knee leg raises

odyforlife.com   www.bodyforlife.com   www.bodyforlife.com   www.bodyforlife.com   www.bodyforlife.com   www.bodyforlife.co

Major Muscle Groups

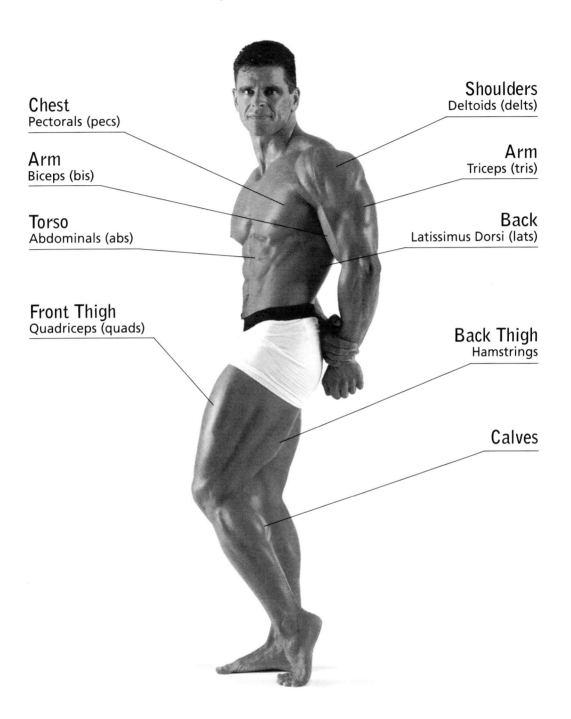

Chest
Pectorals (pecs)

Arm
Biceps (bis)

Torso
Abdominals (abs)

Front Thigh
Quadriceps (quads)

Shoulders
Deltoids (delts)

Arm
Triceps (tris)

Back
Latissimus Dorsi (lats)

Back Thigh
Hamstrings

Calves

w.bodyforlife.com   www.bodyforlife.com   www.bodyforlife.com   www.bodyforlife.com   **www.bodyforlife.com**   www.bodyforlif

Dumbbell Bench Press (chest)

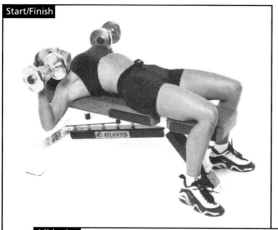

Start/Finish

Starting Position: Lie on your back on a bench, holding a dumbbell in each hand. Bring the weights to a point just above your shoulders, palms facing toward your feet and elbows out.

This is a great chest exercise. I like it even more than the barbell bench press. By using dumbbells, you can stimulate your chest muscles even more, and it's easier on your shoulders.

Midpoint

The Exercise: Press the weights straight up until they're locked out right over your collarbone (not over your face and not over your belly). Then *slowly* lower them to the starting position, feeling the stretch in your chest muscles as your elbows drop below the level of the bench.

This one's a bit awkward at first, but sometimes exercises that feel the most "clumsy" are the ones which work the best.

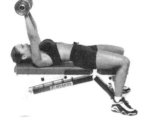

TIP

Don't let the dumbbells sway back toward your head and over your face.

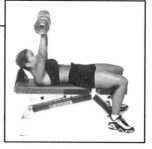

TIP

Don't lift your head off the bench throughout the exercise.

odyforlife.com   www.bodyforlife.com   www.bodyforlife.com   www.bodyforlife.com   www.bodyforlife.com   www.bodyforlife.c

Incline Dumbbell Press (chest)

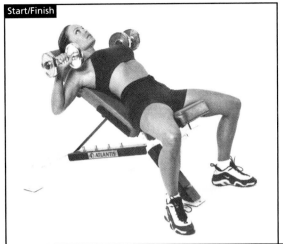

Start/Finish

Starting Position: Sit on the edge of an incline bench. Pick up a dumbbell with each hand, place them on your thighs, and then, one at a time, position them at the base of your shoulders. Lean back, get firmly situated on the bench, and you're ready to go.

Midpoint

The Exercise: Press the weights up to a point over your upper chest, and hold 'em there for a count of one. Then, inhale deeply as you lower the weights to the starting position. Hold the weights in the bottom position for a brief count of one, and then exhale and drive 'em back up.

Because of the angle and leverage, you probably won't be able to lift as much as you can on the flat dumbbell bench press, but that's okay—we're trying to set a record for how much we can improve ourselves; we're *not* trying to set any weight lifting records.

TIP

Don't set your bench at too steep of an incline, or you'll work your shoulders more than your chest.

Exercise Guide

139

Dumbbell Flyes (chest)

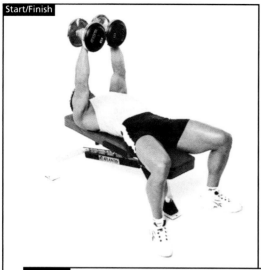

Start/Finish

Midpoint

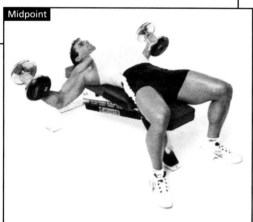

Starting Position: Sit down on the edge of a bench with a dumbbell in each hand. Then lie back, keeping the dumbbells close to your chest. Get firmly situated. Your hips and shoulders stay on the bench, and your feet, flat on the floor.

The Exercise: For the first rep, push the weight up using a pressing-like motion with your palms facing each other. Then, with your elbows slightly bent, slowly lower the dumbbells out to the sides to a point where they are on a horizontal plane even with the bench. Really stretch those pecs, but *don't* try to lower the weights all the way to the floor. Take a count of "I am building my Body-*for*-LIFE" to lower the weights while inhaling deeply.

Once you get to the bottom, hold for a count of one, and then exhale while you lift the weights. Keep your arms stretched out, just slightly bent at the elbows. And move the weights in an arc. Imagine you're wrapping your arms around someone to give them a big hug.

TIP

Don't let your arms go below the level of the bench. This will put too much stress on your shoulders.

bodyforlife.com   www.bodyforlife.com   www.bodyforlife.com   www.bodyforlife.com   www.bodyforlife.com   www.bodyforlife.

Barbell Bench Press (chest)

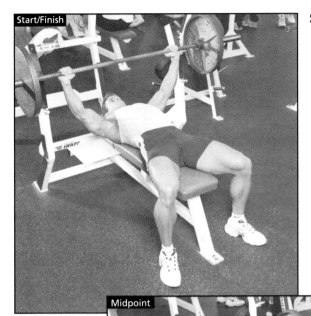

Start/Finish

Midpoint

Starting Position: Lie down on a bench, and firmly position your feet flat on the floor a little more than shoulder width apart. Arch your back slightly, but keep your hips on the bench. Using a grip broader than shoulder width, hold the barbell, with your elbows locked out, right over the middle of your chest.

The Exercise: Start by lowering the weight slowly to a point in the middle of your chest. Make contact with the mid-chest area, pause for a count of one, then, *without* bouncing the barbell off your chest, drive the weight back up. Hold it in the starting position, with your elbows locked out, for another count of one, and repeat.

TIP
Don't lift your hips off the bench while you press the weight up.

Exercise Guide

141

Seated Dumbbell Press (shoulders)

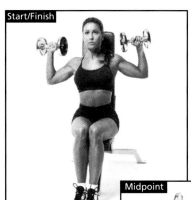

Start/Finish

Midpoint

Starting Position: Sit on the end of a bench with your feet flat on the floor. Hold a dumbbell in each hand, at shoulder height, elbows out, and palms facing forward.

The Exercise: Press the dumbbells up and in, so they nearly touch above your head. Don't let the weights stray back and forth. Press the weights up until your arms are almost straight (your elbows just short of lockout). Then, slowly lower the dumbbells to the starting position.

TIP

Don't lean your head back too far—when doing this exercise, you should look straight forward with your chin up, shoulders squared, and chest high.

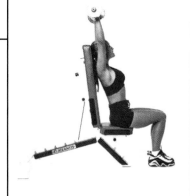

142   Exercise Guide

Standing Barbell Press (shoulders)

Starting Position: Stand with your feet shoulder width apart. Bend your knees slightly, and keep your back straight, not arched. Hold the barbell with a grip just a bit broader than shoulder width apart, right above your collarbone.

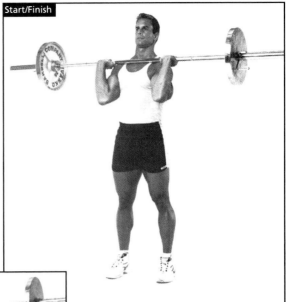

Start/Finish

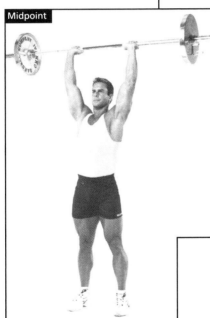

Midpoint

The Exercise: Press the weight up until your arms are fully extended over your head. Pause for a count of one, and then lower the weight slowly to the starting position. Pause at the bottom for, you guessed it, *another* count of one. Do not arch your back as you press the weight overhead on this exercise. That can put undue stress on your lower back.

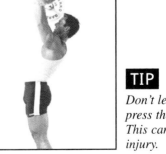

TIP

Don't lean back as you press the weight up. This can cause a back injury.

w.bodyforlife.com   www.bodyforlife.com   www.bodyforlife.com   www.bodyforlife.com   **www.bodyforlife.com**   www.bodyforlife

Side Raises (shoulders)

Starting Position: Stand upright, with your feet about shoulder width apart and your arms at your sides. Hold a dumbbell in each hand, your palms turned toward your body.

It's important to keep your palms turned downward as you lift the dumbbells so your shoulders, rather than your biceps, do the work.

Start/Finish

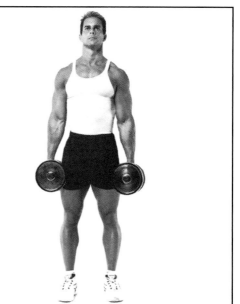

Midpoint

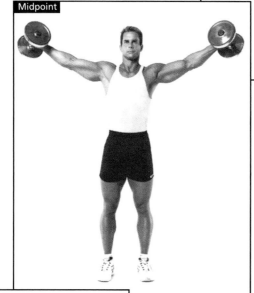

The Exercise: Keeping your arms straight, lift the weights out and up to the sides until they are right about level with your chin, and hold 'em there for a count of one. From this position, lower them slowly back to your sides—remember, there's a lot of good muscle work going on in that portion of the exercise.

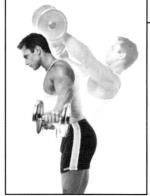

TIP

Don't lean back and "swing" the weights up. Lift them straight out to your sides until they are almost directly out from your shoulders—in the top position, it looks almost like a gymnast doing an iron cross on the rings.

TIP

Don't lean your torso forward and bring the dumbbells down in front of your body. Instead, let the weights down to your sides.

144

Exercise Guide

Bent-Over Raises (shoulders)

Starting Position: With a dumbbell in each hand and your feet shoulder width apart, bend forward at the waist so your upper body is parallel with the floor. Let your arms hang straight down, palms facing each other.

This is a *great* exercise for your rear deltoids (where your back muscles and shoulders come together).

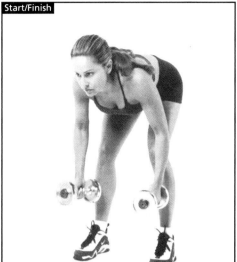

Start/Finish

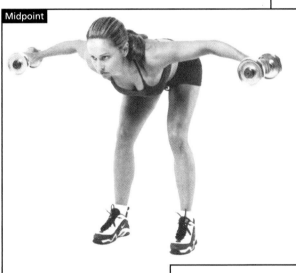

Midpoint

The Exercise: Raise the dumbbells, pulling your arms apart and moving your elbows up. Resist the temptation to raise your torso as you lift the dumbbells. Pause for a count of one at the top when the dumbbells are in line with your shoulders, then slowly lower the weights to the starting position.

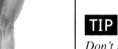

TIP

Don't lean over too much and hunch your back. Your back should be straight, and your torso, almost parallel with the ground.

Exercise Guide

145

Starting Position: Seated on a pulldown machine, position the knee pads so your thighs fit snugly under them. Then firmly grasp a wide bar—your hands should be almost twice your shoulder width apart. This is a great exercise for the major muscles of your back.

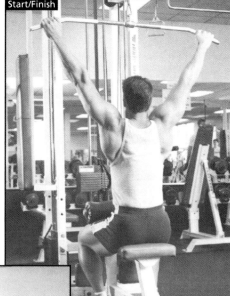

Start/Finish

The Exercise: Pull the bar down to the *top* of your chest. Focus on keeping your elbows directly below the bar. Arch your back slightly, and hold the bar in that position right on top of your collarbone for a count of one; then slowly let the bar back up to the starting position.

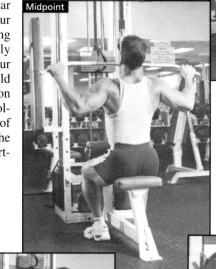

Midpoint

TIP

Don't lean back too far and pull the weight down with momentum.

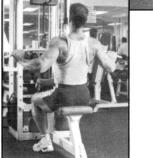

TIP

Don't pull the bar down to your chest bone (sternum). The bar should actually be pulled down to your collarbone area.

bodyforlife.com   www.bodyforlife.com   www.bodyforlife.com   www.bodyforlife.com   www.bodyforlife.com   www.bodyforlife.c

One-Arm Dumbbell Rows (back)

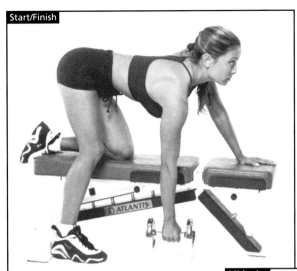

Start/Finish

Starting Position: Start with your right foot flat on the floor and your left knee resting on a flat bench. Then lean forward so you're supporting the weight of your upper body with your left arm on the bench. Your back should be almost parallel with the floor.

Reach down and pick up a dumbbell with your right hand. Look straight ahead instead of at the floor in order to keep your back straight.

The Exercise: Concentrate on pulling your elbow as far back as it can go. The dumbbell should end up roughly parallel with your torso. After you've "rowed" the dumbbell up as far as you can, slowly lower it to the starting position.

After you complete the planned number of reps for your right arm, follow the same instructions for your left.

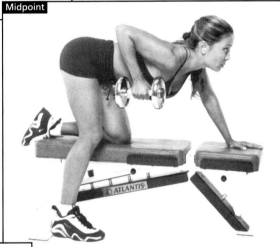

Midpoint

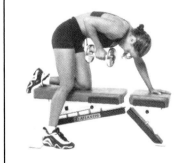

TIP

Don't hunch or round your back. Keep it flat.

w.bodyforlife.com   www.bodyforlife.com   www.bodyforlife.com   www.bodyforlife.com   **www.bodyforlife.com**   www.bodyforlife

Reverse-Grip Pulldowns (back)

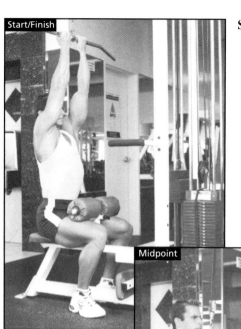

Start/Finish

Midpoint

Starting Position: Seated on a pulldown machine, reach up and take a shoulder-width grip with your palms facing you (hence, the reverse grip).

The Exercise: From this stretched position, pull the bar down to your *upper* chest while contracting your back muscles and keeping your elbows in close to your body. Your back should be arched slightly, your chest high, chin up, and your abs and lower back tight.

Then, let the weight back up, resisting it as you straighten your arms. As you finish the rep, your arms should be fully extended, and your lats will be stretched.

TIP

Don't lean back too far and let momentum take over.

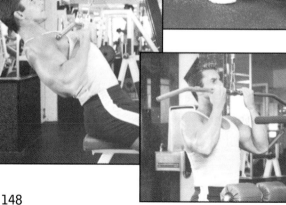

TIP

Remember to pull the bar down all the way to your collarbone—if you just pull it down to your chin, you won't maximize the amount of work your back muscles get.

148

Exercise Guide

Dumbbell Pullovers (back)

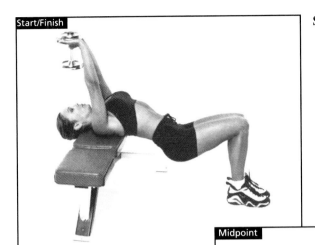

Start/Finish

Starting Position: Lie *across* a flat bench. Be sure only your upper back makes contact with the bench. Lift the weight overhead, and hold it at arm's length over your face.

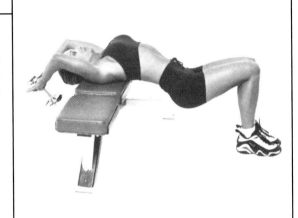

Midpoint

The Exercise: Without raising your hips, lower the dumbbell, in an arc, slowly, while you breathe in *very deeply*. When you reach a fully stretched position, hold it for a quick count of one, and then raise the weight back up, in an arc, and exhale deeply.

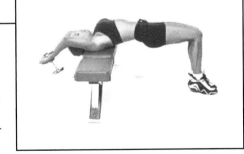

TIP

Don't let your hips rise up as the dumbbell is lowered behind your head—keep your hips in the same low spot.

Exercise Guide

149

Dumbbell Extensions (triceps)

Starting Position: On this exercise, you have to use a dumbbell that has collars which hold the weights on firmly. Stand with your feet shoulder width apart and your knees slightly bent. Grasp one end of a dumbbell with both hands (palms up), and raise it above your head.

The Exercise: Start by bending your arms and slowly lowering the dumbbell behind your head. Keep your elbows close to your head and pointed straight up throughout the exercise to keep the focus on your triceps, not on your shoulders. Lower the weight until you feel a stretch in your triceps, hold for a count of one, and press the weight back up, following an *arc* so you don't bonk the back of your head.

Keep lifting until your arms are locked out and the dumbbell is again directly over your head.

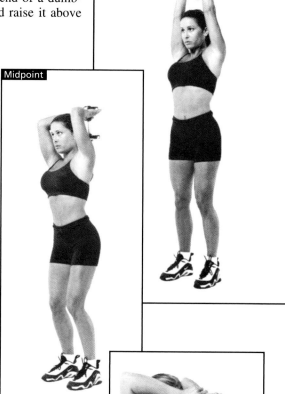

Start/Finish

Midpoint

TIP

Keep your elbows pointed up, and hold them in—don't let them flare out to the sides.

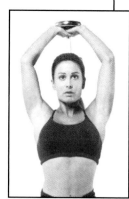

TIP

Don't hold the dumbbell like a sandwich. Place your palms so they face the inside end plate of the dumbbell, with your index fingers and thumbs touching.

odyforlife.com   www.bodyforlife.com   www.bodyforlife.com   www.bodyforlife.com   www.bodyforlife.com   www.bodyforlife.c

Close-Grip Pushdowns (triceps)

Starting Position: Using a high-cable machine, take a slightly closer than shoulder-width, palms-down grip. Position your forearms so they are about parallel with the floor. Keep your feet shoulder width apart for added stability, and bend your knees slightly. Your wrists should be locked in a neutral position (neither bent forward nor back) for the duration of the exercise. Tighten your abdominals to stabilize your upper torso and keep it from swaying. (Got all that?)

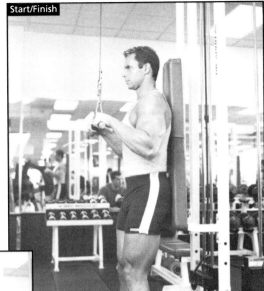

The Exercise: Push the bar down and in toward your legs in a circular motion until your arms are straight and your elbows are locked. Keep your upper arms close to your body, and flex those triceps in the bottom position for a count of one. Then let the weight slowly return to the starting position, and do it again.

TIP

Don't hunch forward and lean over the bar—the proper form should be with your shoulders squared, chest and chin up, and your eyes looking straight forward.

w.bodyforlife.com   www.bodyforlife.com   www.bodyforlife.com   www.bodyforlife.com   **www.bodyforlife.com**   www.bodyforli

Bench Dips (triceps)

Starting Position: Stand with your back to a sturdy bench or chair. Bend your legs and place your hands on the front edge of the bench. Position your feet in front of you so most of your body weight is resting on your arms.

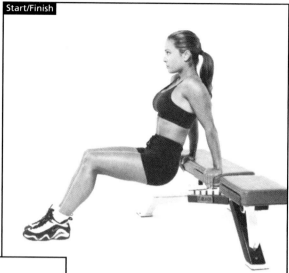

Start/Finish

Midpoint

The Exercise: Keeping your elbows tucked against your sides, bend your arms and slowly lower your body until your upper arms are parallel with the floor. Your hips should drop straight down. Then, straighten your arms to return to the starting position.

TIP

Don't lower your body too far. That can stress your shoulders.

TIP

Don't let your upper body extend too far out away from the bench, which also creates stress on your shoulder joints. Your hips should stay pretty close to the bench.

152

Exercise Guide

Lying Dumbbell Extensions (triceps)

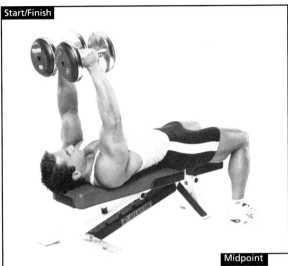

Start/Finish

Starting Position: Lie down on a flat bench with a dumbbell in each hand, arms extended over your head, so you are looking straight up at them. Your palms should be facing each other.

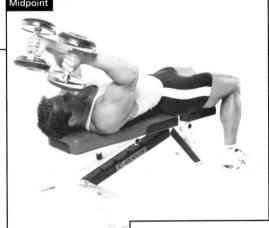

Midpoint

The Exercise: Bend your elbows and *slowly* lower the dumbbells toward your shoulders, *not* toward your head. Your upper arms should remain stationary. Keep your elbows pointed *up*, not back.

This is a great triceps exercise, but it's hard at first. Keep practicing, and you'll get the hang of it.

TIP

Don't let your elbows flare out. Keep them in and pointed straight up.

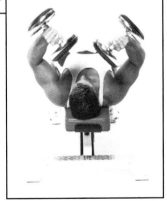

v.bodyforlife.com   www.bodyforlife.com   www.bodyforlife.com   www.bodyforlife.com   **www.bodyforlife.com**   www.bodyforlife

Incline Dumbbell Curls (biceps)

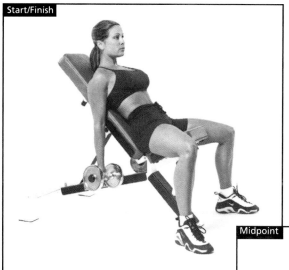

Start/Finish

Starting Position: Grab a pair of dumbbells, and sit down on an incline bench. Keep your shoulders squared and your chest elevated. In the starting position, your arms will be hanging straight down.

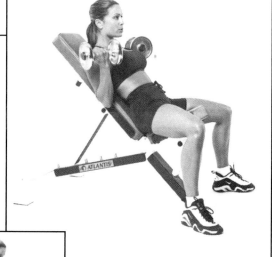

Midpoint

The Exercise: While keeping your back flat against the bench and your palms facing *forward*, curl the dumbbells all the way up to your shoulders. Then slowly lower the weights until your arms are hanging straight down, so you get a full stretch on your biceps before you lift the dumbbells back up.

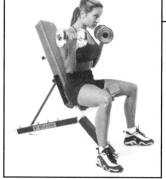

TIP

Don't lean forward away from the back of the incline bench. This usually leads to swinging the weights up.

bodyforlife.com   www.bodyforlife.com   www.bodyforlife.com   www.bodyforlife.com   www.bodyforlife.com   www.bodyforlife.c

Seated Dumbbell Curls (biceps)

Starting Position: Sit on the edge of a flat bench with your arms at your sides, a dumbbell in each hand. Now get ready to focus on flexing your biceps—take a deep breath and begin.

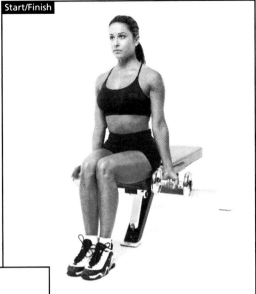

Start/Finish

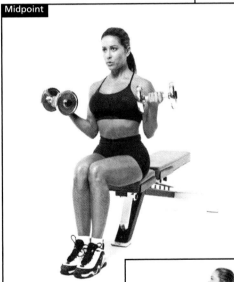

Midpoint

The Exercise: With your palms facing forward, curl both arms, lifting the dumbbells toward your shoulders. During the curl, keep your upper arms and torso still—there will be some movement, but avoid swinging the weight up (a *common* mistake). Let your biceps do the work. Then lower the dumbbells slowly to the starting point.

TIP

Don't lean back or forward as you lower the weights. This cuts down on the amount of work the biceps are doing.

Standing Barbell Curls (biceps)

Starting Position: Stand with your feet roughly shoulder width apart, holding a barbell with a shoulder-width grip. Keep your chest up and shoulders squared—sort of as if you were standing at attention.

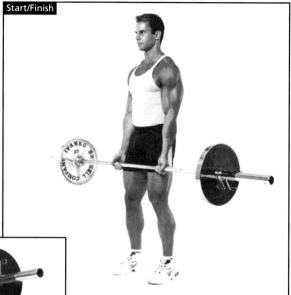

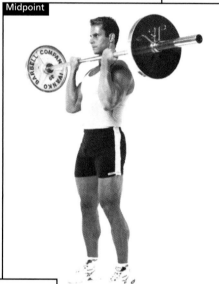

The Exercise: Now, *without* leaning back, curl the weight up, keeping your upper arms close to your sides. Your elbows shouldn't dig into your ribs for leverage, nor should they turn outward. Lower the weight all the way, in a controlled manner.

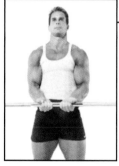

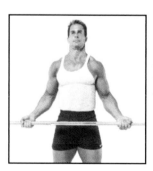

TIP

Don't take a very narrow or very wide grip. Both can cause stress to the wrists and elbows. Your hands should be shoulder width apart.

Exercise Guide

Hammer Curls (biceps)

Starting Position: Stand with your feet roughly shoulder width apart, with your arms extended down at your sides, a dumbbell in each hand, with your palms *facing* each other.

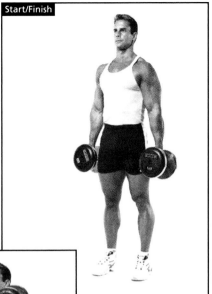

Start/Finish

The Exercise: Curl both arms, lifting the dumbbells toward your shoulders. During the curl, keep your upper arms and torso still. Lower the dumbbells under control. Remember to follow the cadence "I am building my Body-*for*-LIFE."

Because you keep your palms facing each other on this exercise, it works a different part of your upper arms.

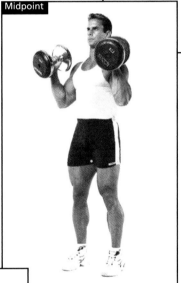

Midpoint

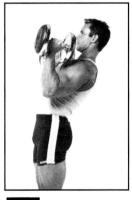

TIP
Don't lean forward or back too much. Keep your abs tight and your torso upright throughout the exercise.

TIP
Don't lift with your palms facing down. The proper form to lift the dumbbells is with your palms facing each other.

.bodyforlife.com   www.bodyforlife.com   www.bodyforlife.com   www.bodyforlife.com   **www.bodyforlife.com**   www.bodyforlife

Leg Extensions (quadriceps)

Starting Position: Sit down on a leg-extension machine, and hook your ankles behind the roller pad. If the roller pad is adjustable, it should be positioned so it rests on the lowest part of your shins, *not* on the top of your feet nor on the middle of your shins. Grasp the handles on the machine or the edges of the seat lightly to keep your hips from lifting up as you perform the exercise.

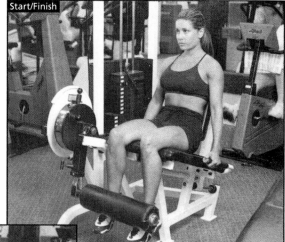
Start/Finish

Midpoint

The Exercise: Straighten your legs, lifting the weight with your quads until your knees are straight. Always try for the fullest range of motion you can—all the way up, all the way down. Remember, we actually *stretch* while we're working out with this Program.

TIP

Lower the weight all the way down—a lot of people go only halfway down and then lift the weight back up. This makes the exercise half *as effective.*

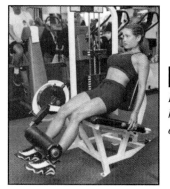

TIP

Don't let your hips come up off the seat.

158

Exercise Guide

Leg Press (quadriceps)

Starting Position: Position yourself on the seat of a leg-press machine, placing your feet about shoulder width apart, toes slightly pointed out on the pressing platform.

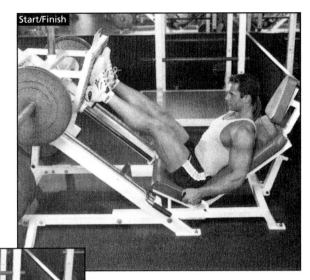

Start/Finish

Midpoint

The Exercise: Slowly lower the weight to a point where your quads touch your belly as you inhale deeply. Then press the weight back to the starting position.

Be sure to push from your heels, *not* your toes, and don't quite lock your knees at the top. This is a great leg exercise, but it is a challenging one.

TIP

Don't put your feet too far apart and point your toes out at a sharp angle. Keep your toes just slightly pointed out, with your feet just about shoulder width apart.

.bodyforlife.com   www.bodyforlife.com   www.bodyforlife.com   www.bodyforlife.com   **www.bodyforlife.com**   www.bodyforlife

Barbell Squats (quadriceps)

Starting Position: Position the barbell on the upper portion of your back, *not* your neck. Firmly grip the bar with your hands almost double shoulder width apart. Position your feet, angled *slightly* out, about shoulder width apart.

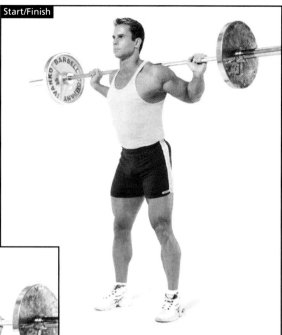

Start/Finish

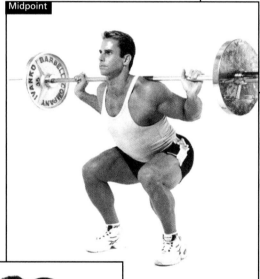

Midpoint

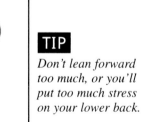

The Exercise: Bend your knees and slowly lower your hips straight down until your thighs are parallel with the floor. Keep your back as straight as possible, your chin up, and your shoulders squared. Once you reach the bottom position, press from your heels, and drive the weight upward. Inhale deeply on the descent, and exhale on the way up. (If you have trouble balancing on this exercise, try placing a sturdy, one-inch-thick wooden block under your heels.)

This is one of the most *demanding* exercises there is, but it works great for building firm, strong legs.

TIP
Don't lean forward too much, or you'll put too much stress on your lower back.

160

Exercise Guide

Dumbbell Squats (quadriceps)

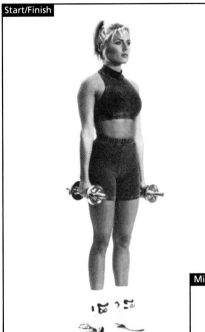

Start/Finish

Starting Position: Hold two dumbbells at your sides, with your palms facing in. Stand with your feet about shoulder width apart. If you have trouble balancing, try placing a sturdy, one-inch-thick wooden block or a couple of dumbbell plates under your heels.

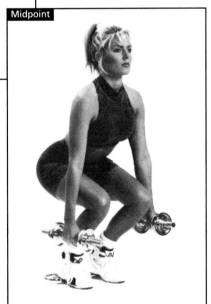

Midpoint

The Exercise: While keeping your shoulders, back, and head upright, bend your legs at the knees and lower your hips until your thighs are parallel with the floor. Then, pushing from your heels, lift yourself back up to the starting position. Keep your back as straight as possible throughout this exercise.

Dumbbell Lunges (hamstrings)

Starting Position: Stand with your feet together, toes pointed straight forward, and a dumbbell in each hand. Keep your shoulders squared, your chin up, and back straight.

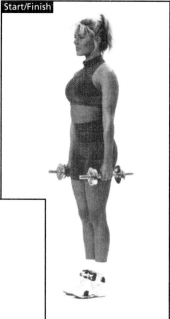

Start/Finish

The Exercise: Step forward with your right foot. Bend at your knees, and lower your hips until your left knee is just a few inches off the floor. Push with the right leg, raising yourself back up to the starting point. Repeat until you've done the planned number of reps for your right leg; then do the same for your left leg.

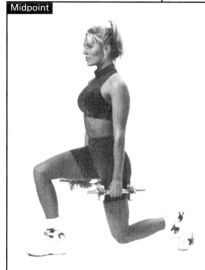

Midpoint

TIP

Don't point your toes in or out. Both feet should point straight forward.

TIP

Don't lift your foot up. Keep it flat. The proper form is with one leg extended to the point where, when you bend down, your knee on the forward leg is over your foot, not way out in front of it.

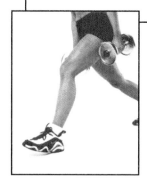

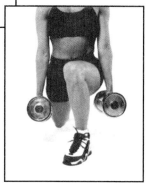

Exercise Guide

Standing Leg Curls (hamstrings)

Starting Position: Using a standing leg curl machine, position your thighs and chest against the pads and your ankle against the roller pad. Lean forward, and grasp the handles.

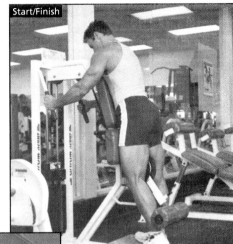
Start/Finish

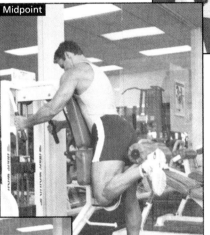
Midpoint

The Exercise: Curl the weight up, flex your hamstring (the back of your leg) as hard as you can, and hold it for a count of one. Then *slowly* lower the weight all the way down to the starting position. After you've finished the planned number of reps with one leg, do the same for your opposite leg.

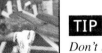
TIP

Don't lean forward or stick your hips way out. On this exercise, your whole body should be straight.

Exercise Guide

163

Lying Leg Curls (hamstrings)

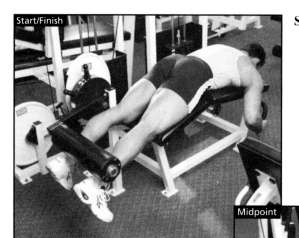

Start/Finish

Starting Position: Lie facedown on a lying leg curl machine, adjusting your position so the pads are resting on the back of your ankles.

Midpoint

The Exercise: Curl your legs up, and bring your feet as close to your hips as possible; ideally, the roller pad should touch the top of your hamstrings. Hold this fully contracted position for a count of one before *slowly* lowering the weight to the starting position, once again trying for the full range of motion.

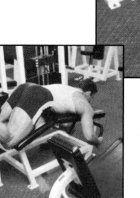

TIP
Don't lift your hips as you curl the weight as this puts stress on your lower back.

bodyforlife.com   www.bodyforlife.com   www.bodyforlife.com   www.bodyforlife.com   www.bodyforlife.com   www.bodyforlife.c

Straight-Leg Deadlifts (hamstrings)

Start/Finish

Starting Position: Stand up straight, with your feet shoulder width apart and a dumbbell in each hand, your palms facing toward your legs.

This is a terrific exercise for the hamstrings, and it helps strengthen the lower back.

The Exercise: Bend forward at your hips, and slowly lower the dumbbells in front of you until the weights almost touch the floor. Keep your back straight throughout the exercise. Then, while concentrating on the muscles in the back of your legs, raise your upper body and the weights to the starting position.

Midpoint

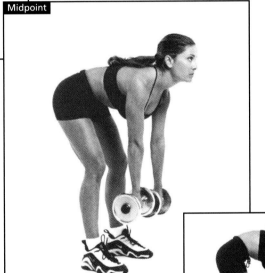

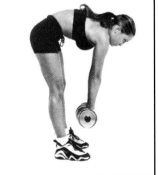

TIP

Don't hunch over. Keep your back fairly rigid throughout the exercise.

w.bodyforlife.com   www.bodyforlife.com   www.bodyforlife.com   www.bodyforlife.com   **www.bodyforlife.com**   www.bodyforlif

Seated Calf Raises (calves)

Starting Position: Position yourself on a seated calf-raise machine with the balls of your feet on the platform and the knee pad on the lower part of your front thigh. Keep your upper body still during the exercise, and focus on those calves.

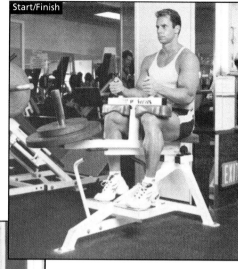

Start/Finish

Midpoint

The Exercise: Slowly lower your heels and let your calf muscles stretch as far down as you can. Hold that stretch for a count of one before pressing the weight up as high as possible. Flex hard and hold for another count of one. Then lower the weight slowly.

TIP

Don't put the pads high up on your thighs. The pad should be placed down closer to your knees.

bodyforlife.com   www.bodyforlife.com   www.bodyforlife.com   www.bodyforlife.com   www.bodyforlife.com   www.bodyforlife.c

Standing Calf Raises (calves)

Starting Position: Using, you guessed it . . . a standing calf-raise machine, position yourself so the balls of your feet are on the platform and the pads which transfer the weight are on top of your shoulders. Don't hunch over.

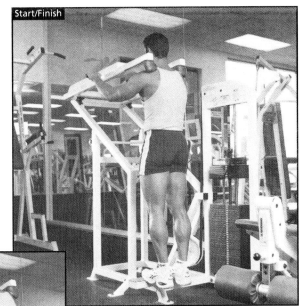

Start/Finish

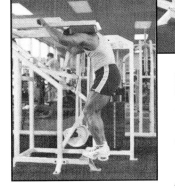

Midpoint

The Exercise: Without bending at your hips or knees, slowly lower the weight, using a count of "I am building my Body-*for*-LIFE," and stretch your calf muscles as far as you can. Hold them in that lower position for a count of one. Then lift the weight up as high as you can, and hold the contraction for another count of one.

TIP

Don't let your back hunch over. Keep your shoulders squared, your chin up, and your face forward.

Exercise Guide

167

One-Leg Calf Raise (calves)

Start/Finish

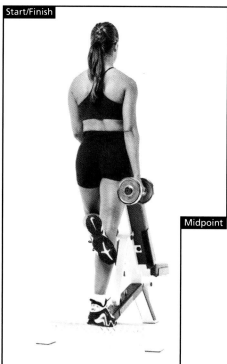

Starting Position: Stand with the ball of your right foot resting on a step or a sturdy wooden block, a dumbbell in your right hand, holding on to something for balance with your left hand. Lift your left foot up and hook it behind your right calf.

Midpoint

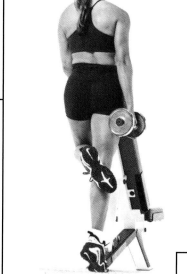

The Exercise: Lower your right heel as far as you can, really stretching your calf at the bottom. Then press up on your toes as far as possible, contracting the calf muscle. Hold that flex for a count of one; then slowly lower the weight, and repeat for the planned number of reps. Switch legs, and follow the same instructions.

TIP

Don't let your foot roll toward the little toe when you're lifting. Instead, raise up, flexing your calf, and put the weight on the ball of your foot.

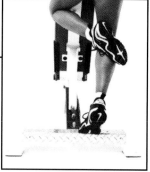

168   Exercise Guide

Angled Calf Raise (calves)

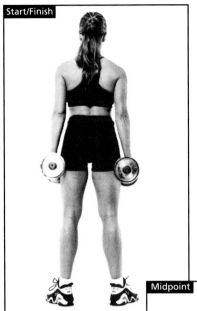

Start/Finish

Starting Position: This is a good calf exercise you can do at home or at a gym. All you need is a pair of dumbbells. Start by holding a dumbbell in each hand and standing with your feet about shoulder width apart. Now, turn your toes out, so your feet form a 45-degree angle.

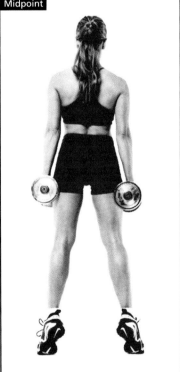

Midpoint

The Exercise: Keeping your legs straight, raise up on your toes as high as possible. Pause for a count of one, then slowly lower to the starting position.

TIP

Don't do this exercise on carpet—find a solid surface like a hard-wood or concrete floor.

w.bodyforlife.com   www.bodyforlife.com   www.bodyforlife.com   www.bodyforlife.com   **www.bodyforlife.com**   www.bodyforlife

Floor Crunches (abdominals)

Starting Position: Of all the newfangled doodads and gimmick devices that promise to deliver a firm, "sexy" tummy in record time, I'm convinced none work as well as a properly executed, simple abdominal-strengthening exercise called floor crunches.

All you do is lie on a floor (preferably a carpeted floor or a pad of some kind), put your hands beside your head, bring your knees together, and place your feet flat on the floor about a foot from your hips.

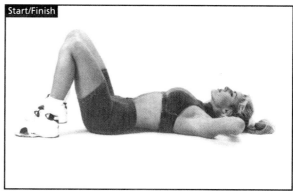

Start/Finish

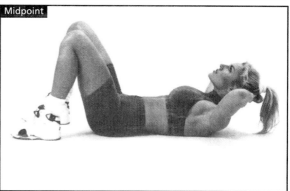

Midpoint

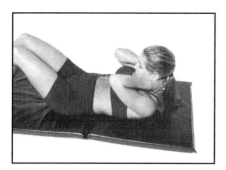

TIP

Don't lock your hands behind your head. Your hands should be cupped at the sides of your head and should not be used for leverage.

The Exercise: Start by pushing your lower back down, almost like you're trying to make a dent in the floor. Then and only then, begin to roll your shoulders up, keeping your knees and hips stationary. Continue to push down as hard as you can with your lower back.

The range of motion on this exercise is very limited. Your shoulders actually come off the ground only a few inches. Hold this position and flex your abdominal muscles as hard as you can for a count of one, and then slowly lower your shoulders back down to the floor, but never stop pushing down with your lower back.

Take your time on this exercise. It's not a race, and it's not a contest to see who can do the most sit-ups. If you do this exercise properly, I guarantee your abs will be burning by the time you get done with a dozen reps.

bodyforlife.com   **www.bodyforlife.com**   www.bodyforlife.com   www.bodyforlife.com   www.bodyforlife.com   www.bodyforlife.c

Twist Crunches (abdominals)

Starting Position: Lie flat on your back with your knees bent and your hands beside your head. Let your legs fall as far as they can to your left side so your upper body is flat on the floor and your lower body is on its side.

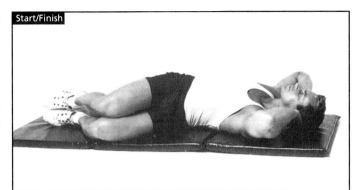

Start/Finish

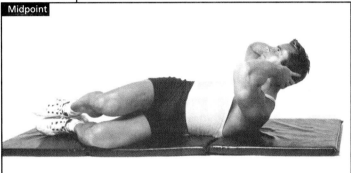

Midpoint

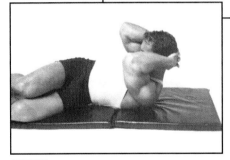

TIP

Don't lock your hands behind your head.

The Exercise: Press your lower back down into the floor, while you roll your upper body slightly up until your shoulder blades clear the ground. Concentrate on the obliques (the muscles on the sides of your waist), and contract and hold the crunch for a count of one. The key to making this exercise ultra-effective is to hold that contraction. (Most people don't do this—they simply lift up and then lower back down.)

After you've held that contraction, slowly lower to the starting position, count one, then perform your next rep. After you complete the planned number of reps on the right side, switch to your left and follow the same instructions.

v.bodyforlife.com   www.bodyforlife.com   www.bodyforlife.com   www.bodyforlife.com   **www.bodyforlife.com**   www.bodyforlife

Decline Sit-Ups (abdominals)

Starting Position: This is a great exercise for the lower and middle abs.

In order to do this one, you'll need a "decline bench" that allows you to hook your feet. Position yourself on the decline bench with your feet locked in. Your upper body should be perpendicular to the bench, so you have to contract your abs just to remain in place. Place your hands on each side of your head, just behind your ears. Don't lock your fingers.

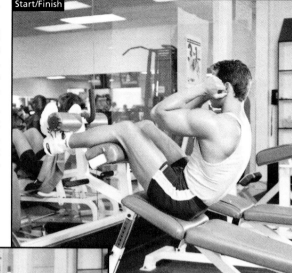

Start/Finish

Midpoint

The Exercise: Lower your upper body while you contract your abs. Go back just about a foot. (Do *not* go all the way down.) Hold and flex extra hard for a count of one. Then crunch back up to the starting position. When your strength increases and you can do more than 12 reps, grab a weight plate (start with just 10 pounds) and perform the exercise as described here, while holding the weight against your chest.

TIP
Don't go back too far—this will put stress on your lower back.

bodyforlife.com   www.bodyforlife.com   www.bodyforlife.com   www.bodyforlife.com   www.bodyforlife.com   www.bodyforlife.c

Bent-Knee Leg Raises (abdominals)

Starting Position: Lie flat on your back on a padded or carpeted floor with your hands under your hips, palms down for support. Lift your head slightly off the floor, but don't bring your chin to your chest.

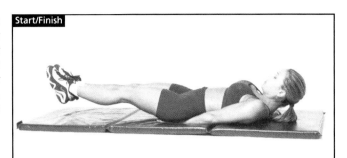

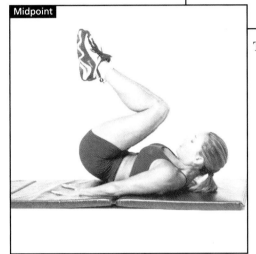

The Exercise: Start by lifting your legs off the floor while you simultaneously bend them at your knees, pulling your thighs up toward your chest, slowly. Now, with your knees approaching your chest, contract your abs and slightly lift your pelvis up off the floor.

Then, slowly straighten your legs. Bring them back down toward the floor, but *don't* let them rest on the floor. Hold them in that extended position for a count of one, and then bring 'em back up.

TIP

Don't lift your head up too far or let your lower back arch; your lower back should be pressed into the ground, and your head should stay back, just slightly off the ground.

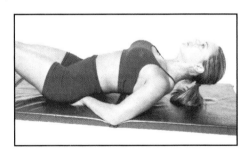

Notice: If you'd like to see a video demonstration of any of the exercises shown in this section, visit www.bodyforlife.com.

w.bodyforlife.com   www.bodyforlife.com   www.bodyforlife.com   www.bodyforlife.com   **www.bodyforlife.com**   www.bodyforlife

Daily Progress Reports

Appendix D

w.bodyforlife.com   www.bodyforlife.com   www.bodyforlife.com   www.bodyforlife.com   **www.bodyforlife.com**   www.bodyforlife

The Eating-*for*-LIFE Method
Daily Progress Report

Date:	Day 1 of 84

Total portions of protein: 6	Total portions of protein:
Total portions of carbs: 6	Total portions of carbs:
Total cups of water: 10	Total cups of water:

PLAN	ACTUAL
Meal 1 ☐ a.m. ☐ p.m.	**Meal 1** ☐ a.m. ☐ p.m.
Meal 2 ☐ a.m. ☐ p.m.	**Meal 2** ☐ a.m. ☐ p.m.
Meal 3 ☐ a.m. ☐ p.m.	**Meal 3** ☐ a.m. ☐ p.m.
Meal 4 ☐ a.m. ☐ p.m.	**Meal 4** ☐ a.m. ☐ p.m.
Meal 5 ☐ a.m. ☐ p.m.	**Meal 5** ☐ a.m. ☐ p.m.
Meal 6 ☐ a.m. ☐ p.m.	**Meal 6** ☐ a.m. ☐ p.m.

NOTES

bodyforlife.com   www.bodyforlife.com   www.bodyforlife.com   www.bodyforlife.com   www.bodyforlife.com   www.bodyforlife.c

The Training-*for*-LIFE Experience™
Daily Progress Report

Intensity Pattern

Date:	Planned Start Time:	Actual Start Time:
Day 1 of 84	Planned End Time:	Actual End Time:
Upper Body Workout	Time to Complete: 46 minutes	Total Time:

Upper Body Muscle Groups	Exercise	PLAN				ACTUAL			
		Reps	Weight (lbs)	Minutes Between Sets	Intensity Level	Reps	Weight (lbs)	Minutes Between Sets	Intensity Level
Chest		12		1	5				
		10		1	6				
		8		1	7				
		6		1	8				
High Point		12		0	9				
		12		2	10				
Shoulders		12		1	5				
		10		1	6				
		8		1	7				
		6		1	8				
High Point		12		0	9				
		12		2	10				
Back		12		1	5				
		10		1	6				
		8		1	7				
		6		1	8				
High Point		12		0	9				
		12		2	10				
Triceps		12		1	5				
		10		1	6				
		8		1	7				
		6		1	8				
High Point		12		0	9				
		12		2	10				

At this point, you should be 37 minutes into your upper body weight-training workout and have 9 minutes to go.

Biceps		12		1	5				
		10		1	6				
		8		1	7				
		6		1	8				
High Point		12		0	9				
		12		–	10				

NOTES

---

www.bodyforlife.com   www.bodyforlife.com   www.bodyforlife.com   www.bodyforlife.com   **www.bodyforlife.com**   www.bodyforlife

The Eating-*for*-LIFE Method
Daily Progress Report

Date:	Day 2 of 84

Total portions of protein: 6	Total portions of protein:
Total portions of carbs: 6	Total portions of carbs:
Total cups of water: 10	Total cups of water:

PLAN	ACTUAL
Meal 1 ☐ a.m. ☐ p.m.	**Meal 1** ☐ a.m. ☐ p.m.
Meal 2 ☐ a.m. ☐ p.m.	**Meal 2** ☐ a.m. ☐ p.m.
Meal 3 ☐ a.m. ☐ p.m.	**Meal 3** ☐ a.m. ☐ p.m.
Meal 4 ☐ a.m. ☐ p.m.	**Meal 4** ☐ a.m. ☐ p.m.
Meal 5 ☐ a.m. ☐ p.m.	**Meal 5** ☐ a.m. ☐ p.m.
Meal 6 ☐ a.m. ☐ p.m.	**Meal 6** ☐ a.m. ☐ p.m.

NOTES

.bodyforlife.com   www.bodyforlife.com   www.bodyforlife.com   www.bodyforlife.com   www.bodyforlife.com   www.bodyforlife.

The 20-Minute Aerobics Solution™
Daily Progress Report

Intensity Pattern

Date:	Planned Start Time:	Actual Start Time:
Day 2 of 84	Planned End Time:	Actual End Time:
Aerobic Workout	Time to Complete: 20 minutes	Total Time:

Exercise	PLAN		Exercise	ACTUAL	
	Minute by Minute	Intensity Level		Minute by Minute	Intensity Level
	1	5		1	
	2	5		2	
	3	6		3	
	4	7		4	
	5	8		5	
	6	9		6	
	7	6		7	
	8	7		8	
	9	8		9	
	10	9		10	
	11	6		11	
	12	7		12	
	13	8		13	
	14	9		14	
	15	6		15	
	16	7		16	
	17	8		17	
High Point	18	9	**High Point**	18	
	19	10		19	
	20	5		20	

NOTES

_____

_____

_____

_____

Daily Progress Reports

The Eating-*for*-LIFE Method
Daily Progress Report

Body
for
LIFE

Date:	Day 3 of 84

Total portions of protein: 6	Total portions of protein:
Total portions of carbs: 6	Total portions of carbs:
Total cups of water: 10	Total cups of water:

PLAN	ACTUAL
Meal 1 ☐ a.m. ☐ p.m.	**Meal 1** ☐ a.m. ☐ p.m.
Meal 2 ☐ a.m. ☐ p.m.	**Meal 2** ☐ a.m. ☐ p.m.
Meal 3 ☐ a.m. ☐ p.m.	**Meal 3** ☐ a.m. ☐ p.m.
Meal 4 ☐ a.m. ☐ p.m.	**Meal 4** ☐ a.m. ☐ p.m.
Meal 5 ☐ a.m. ☐ p.m.	**Meal 5** ☐ a.m. ☐ p.m.
Meal 6 ☐ a.m. ☐ p.m.	**Meal 6** ☐ a.m. ☐ p.m.

NOTES

_____

_____

_____

_____

bodyforlife.com   www.bodyforlife.com   www.bodyforlife.com   www.bodyforlife.com   www.bodyforlife.com   www.bodyforlife.c

The Training-*for*-LIFE Experience™
Daily Progress Report

Intensity Pattern

Date:	Planned Start Time:	Actual Start Time:
Day 3 of 84	Planned End Time:	Actual End Time:
Lower Body Workout	Time to Complete: 42 minutes	Total Time:

Lower Body Muscle Groups	Exercise	PLAN				ACTUAL			
		Reps	Weight (lbs)	Minutes Between Sets	Intensity Level	Reps	Weight (lbs)	Minutes Between Sets	Intensity Level
Quads		12		1	5				
		10		1	6				
		8		1	7				
		6		1	8				
High Point		12		0	9				
		12		2	10				
Ham-strings		12		1	5				
		10		1	6				
		8		1	7				
		6		1	8				
High Point		12		0	9				
		12		2	10				
Calves		12		1	5				
		10		1	6				
		8		1	7				
		6		1	8				
High Point		12		0	9				
		12		2	10				

At this point, you should be 31 minutes into your lower body weight-training workout and have 11 minutes to go.

Abs		12		1	5				
		10		1	6				
		8		1	7				
		6		1	8				
High Point		12		0	9				
		12		–	10				

NOTES

_____

_____

_____

_____

Daily Progress Reports

181

The Eating-*for*-LIFE Method
Daily Progress Report

Date:	Day 4 of 84

Total portions of protein: 6	Total portions of protein:
Total portions of carbs: 6	Total portions of carbs:
Total cups of water: 10	Total cups of water:

PLAN	ACTUAL
Meal 1 ☐ a.m. ☐ p.m.	**Meal 1** ☐ a.m. ☐ p.m.
Meal 2 ☐ a.m. ☐ p.m.	**Meal 2** ☐ a.m. ☐ p.m.
Meal 3 ☐ a.m. ☐ p.m.	**Meal 3** ☐ a.m. ☐ p.m.
Meal 4 ☐ a.m. ☐ p.m.	**Meal 4** ☐ a.m. ☐ p.m.
Meal 5 ☐ a.m. ☐ p.m.	**Meal 5** ☐ a.m. ☐ p.m.
Meal 6 ☐ a.m. ☐ p.m.	**Meal 6** ☐ a.m. ☐ p.m.

NOTES

odyforlife.com   www.bodyforlife.com   www.bodyforlife.com   www.bodyforlife.com   www.bodyforlife.com   www.bodyforlife.co

Date:	Planned Start Time:	Actual Start Time:
Day 4 of 84	Planned End Time:	Actual End Time:
Aerobic Workout	Time to Complete: 20 minutes	Total Time:

Exercise	PLAN		Exercise	ACTUAL	
	Minute by Minute	Intensity Level		Minute by Minute	Intensity Level
	1	5		1	
	2	5		2	
	3	6		3	
	4	7		4	
	5	8		5	
	6	9		6	
	7	6		7	
	8	7		8	
	9	8		9	
	10	9		10	
	11	6		11	
	12	7		12	
	13	8		13	
	14	9		14	
	15	6		15	
	16	7		16	
	17	8		17	
High Point	18	9	High Point	18	
	19	10		19	
	20	5		20	

NOTES

_____

_____

_____

_____

Daily Progress Reports

The Eating-*for*-LIFE Method
Daily Progress Report

Body
for
LIFE

Date:	Day 5 of 84

Total portions of protein: 6	Total portions of protein:
Total portions of carbs: 6	Total portions of carbs:
Total cups of water: 10	Total cups of water:

PLAN	ACTUAL
Meal 1 ☐ a.m. ☐ p.m.	**Meal 1** ☐ a.m. ☐ p.m.
Meal 2 ☐ a.m. ☐ p.m.	**Meal 2** ☐ a.m. ☐ p.m.
Meal 3 ☐ a.m. ☐ p.m.	**Meal 3** ☐ a.m. ☐ p.m.
Meal 4 ☐ a.m. ☐ p.m.	**Meal 4** ☐ a.m. ☐ p.m.
Meal 5 ☐ a.m. ☐ p.m.	**Meal 5** ☐ a.m. ☐ p.m.
Meal 6 ☐ a.m. ☐ p.m.	**Meal 6** ☐ a.m. ☐ p.m.

NOTES

odyforlife.com www.bodyforlife.com www.bodyforlife.com www.bodyforlife.com www.bodyforlife.com www.bodyforlife.co

The Training-*for*-LIFE Experience™
Daily Progress Report

Intensity Pattern

Date:	Planned Start Time:	Actual Start Time:
Day 5 of 84	Planned End Time:	Actual End Time:
Upper Body Workout	Time to Complete: 46 minutes	Total Time:

Upper Body Muscle Groups	Exercise	PLAN				ACTUAL			
		Reps	Weight (lbs)	Minutes Between Sets	Intensity Level	Reps	Weight (lbs)	Minutes Between Sets	Intensity Level
Chest		12		1	5				
		10		1	6				
		8		1	7				
		6		1	8				
High Point		12		0	9				
		12		2	10				
Shoulders		12		1	5				
		10		1	6				
		8		1	7				
		6		1	8				
High Point		12		0	9				
		12		2	10				
Back		12		1	5				
		10		1	6				
		8		1	7				
		6		1	8				
High Point		12		0	9				
		12		2	10				
Triceps		12		1	5				
		10		1	6				
		8		1	7				
		6		1	8				
High Point		12		0	9				
		12		2	10				

At this point, you should be 37 minutes into your upper body weight-training workout and have 9 minutes to go.

Upper Body Muscle Groups	Exercise	Reps	Weight (lbs)	Minutes Between Sets	Intensity Level	Reps	Weight (lbs)	Minutes Between Sets	Intensity Level
Biceps		12		1	5				
		10		1	6				
		8		1	7				
		6		1	8				
High Point		12		0	9				
		12		–	10				

NOTES

w.bodyforlife.com   www.bodyforlife.com   www.bodyforlife.com   www.bodyforlife.com   **www.bodyforlife.com**   www.bodyforlife

The Eating-*for*-LIFE Method
Daily Progress Report

Date:	Day 6 of 84

Total portions of protein: 6	Total portions of protein:
Total portions of carbs: 6	Total portions of carbs:
Total cups of water: 10	Total cups of water:

PLAN	ACTUAL
Meal 1 ☐ a.m. ☐ p.m.	**Meal 1** ☐ a.m. ☐ p.m.
Meal 2 ☐ a.m. ☐ p.m.	**Meal 2** ☐ a.m. ☐ p.m.
Meal 3 ☐ a.m. ☐ p.m.	**Meal 3** ☐ a.m. ☐ p.m.
Meal 4 ☐ a.m. ☐ p.m.	**Meal 4** ☐ a.m. ☐ p.m.
Meal 5 ☐ a.m. ☐ p.m.	**Meal 5** ☐ a.m. ☐ p.m.
Meal 6 ☐ a.m. ☐ p.m.	**Meal 6** ☐ a.m. ☐ p.m.

NOTES

bodyforlife.com   www.bodyforlife.com   www.bodyforlife.com   www.bodyforlife.com   www.bodyforlife.com   www.bodyforlife.c

The 20-Minute Aerobics Solution™
Daily Progress Report

Intensity Pattern

Date:	Planned Start Time:	Actual Start Time:
Day 6 of 84	Planned End Time:	Actual End Time:
Aerobic Workout	Time to Complete: 20 minutes	Total Time:

Exercise	PLAN		Exercise	ACTUAL	
	Minute by Minute	Intensity Level		Minute by Minute	Intensity Level
	1	5		1	
	2	5		2	
	3	6		3	
	4	7		4	
	5	8		5	
	6	9		6	
	7	6		7	
	8	7		8	
	9	8		9	
	10	9		10	
	11	6		11	
	12	7		12	
	13	8		13	
	14	9		14	
	15	6		15	
	16	7		16	
	17	8		17	
High Point	18	9	**High Point**	18	
	19	10		19	
	20	5		20	

NOTES

_____

_____

_____

_____

w.bodyforlife.com   www.bodyforlife.com   www.bodyforlife.com   www.bodyforlife.com   **www.bodyforlife.com**   www.bodyforlife

Real-Life Success Stories

.bodyforlife.com   www.bodyforlife.com   www.bodyforlife.com   www.bodyforlife.com   **www.bodyforlife.com**   www.bodyforlife

"I've reached a new level of physical and mental fitness."

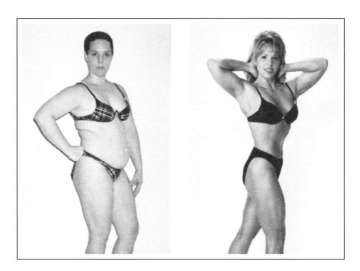

It was early last year when I found out my mother was terminally ill with cancer. When I was told she had only three months to live, I was devastated. I moved from California, where I was living at the time, to Florida, to help my sister take care of her.

My mom and I have always been close. Seeing her sick and bedridden tore me apart. I began venting the stress by eating uncontrollably, which made it harder to do the things for her that I wanted. The weight I was gaining left me so weak and exhausted that it became a struggle to make it through each day with any energy at all.

One day I was sitting on the bed with my mom, and I saw our reflections in a mirror. I saw someone dying, but it was *me*, not Mom. It was then I decided I had to change. How could I take care of Mom if I couldn't even take care of myself?

I also realized that my poor condition was hurting her—she didn't want to see me like this. Like all moms, she wanted the best out of life for me. That was it. I had more than enough reasons to accept Bill's challenge.

Since my mother required 24-hour care, time was my biggest constraint. But I was determined. And as the weeks went by, time became less of a problem because I gained back my energy and was able to get so much more done. My friends and family began complimenting me on my appearance and asked me how they could achieve the same extraordinary results. My self-esteem and confidence skyrocketed. After 12 weeks, I was so excited I kept on going! I've lost over 30 pounds, and I'm still making progress. And my mother received the gift I wanted to give her most of all, which was the best I had to give.

Gail Gosselin
Age 32
Marketing Representative; Dade City, Florida

.bodyforlife.com   **www.bodyforlife.com**   www.bodyforlife.com   www.bodyforlife.com   www.bodyforlife.com   www.bodyforlife.c

*"During the process of re-creation,
I realized my purpose in life."*

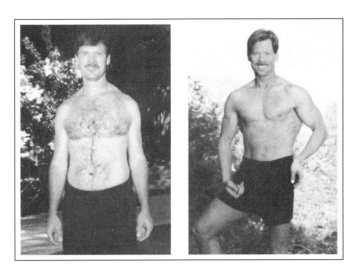

Like many baby boomers, I was dreaming about the day I could retire. I should have been happy this day was in sight for me, but I was miserable. I had spent years training to become an ER doctor. Outwardly, I had it made. I have a great family, my kids are going to the best school in town, and I live in a house bigger than I need. But on the inside, I was miserable. I resented the very things that got me where I was, my mind was stagnant, and my body was on its way to the grave. By accepting mediocrity and giving up hope, I lost my passion for life.

One thing I secretly wished for was to be in exceptional shape. Not overwhelmingly muscular but strong and fit enough to feel good about myself and feel like I was in the "flow" when playing outdoors (mountain biking, hiking, or kayaking). So, I accepted Bill's challenge. My goal was to build my body and find my passion for life again, all in 12 weeks.

The Program was difficult at first, but within a few weeks, I began to feel my confidence and self-esteem rise. My energy level surged, and I was starting to sleep better than I had in a long time. My mind was becoming more acute, and I was interested in the world again.

I reached my physical goals, and I rediscovered passion in my life—my mind, my body, and my soul are one. I am no longer a 47-year-old dreaming of escape. I feel good, I look better, and there is no mountain too high for me to climb.

And, most important of all, during this process of re-creation, which I have gone through over the last 12 weeks, I realized my highest purpose in life is helping others. I can't think of a more gratifying reward.

Russell Simpson, M.D.
Age 47
Physician; Huntsville, Alabama

w.bodyforlife.com   www.bodyforlife.com   www.bodyforlife.com   www.bodyforlife.com   **www.bodyforlife.com**   www.bodyforlife

"We learned how fitness affects every aspect of life."

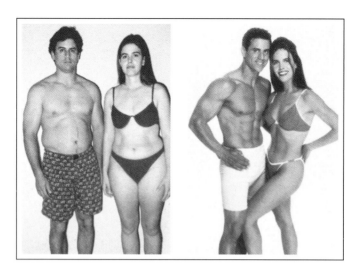

There are moments that mark your life. Moments when you realize nothing will ever be the same, and time is divided into two parts—before this and after this. This Program creates such a moment by providing an opportunity for people of any age, race, or gender to change the way they are living and become healthier, happier, stronger, and more confident.

Over the last few years, our lives had fallen into a rut. We knew nothing about nutrition, worked out very little, and were each about 30 pounds overweight. Worst of all, our self-esteems were plummeting.

We decided to accept Bill's challenge. We set goals as a couple that we would each lose fat, gain muscle, and, for once in our lives, show others that anything is possible.

Little by little, we started to rebuild our physiques, and as our bodies started to strengthen, so did our family. We were finally doing something of extreme significance together. Our children saw their mom and dad work together to achieve the same goal, and we involved them, so they too became part of something special.

We learned how fitness affects every aspect of life. There is no better way to boost your self-worth than by setting and achieving goals. And what better place to start than with your body? We are committed to sharing our experiences with others and showing how they can reach their true potential.

Fred and Stephanie Morales
Ages 30 and 28
Business Owner and Homemaker; Carlsbad, California

bodyforlife.com   www.bodyforlife.com   www.bodyforlife.com   www.bodyforlife.com   www.bodyforlife.com   www.bodyforlife.c

"I lost 19 pounds of fat, and I'm stronger than I have ever been."

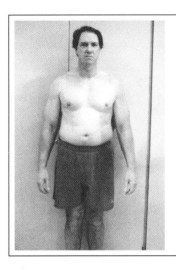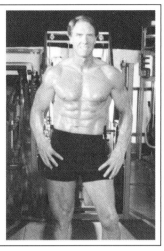

As a teacher and high school football coach, my active lifestyle has always included whatever activities were required to maintain a high level of fitness and a physical appearance I took pride in. However, as I approached my fiftieth birthday, career responsibilities, family commitments, and the rigors of everyday life pushed my plans for personal fitness lower and lower on my priority list. There always seemed to be a reason I couldn't find time to "eat right" or exercise.

Finally, my weight contributed to a chronic back problem and constant pain. And I began to surrender to the tired notion that my best days were behind me and a continual physical decline was all I could look forward to.

I learned about this Program from my doctor while seeking relief from my back pain. As he began to explain the details to me, I had the overwhelming feeling this was the real reason I was there. I was meant to accept this challenge.

Within a few weeks, my muscles began to change and grow almost on a daily basis. They began to become more defined as the layers of fat disappeared. I lost 19 pounds of fat. My back has never felt better. I'm stronger than I have ever been in my life. My cholesterol has dropped to an all-time low.

It is almost as if I have discovered the "secrets of the ages" or the location of the fountain of youth. I feel like I'm 25 again, and my "six-pack" is the envy of every 17-year-old athlete in my high school weight room.

Brandon McFadden
Age 49
Teacher; Oxford, Ohio

v.bodyforlife.com   www.bodyforlife.com   www.bodyforlife.com   www.bodyforlife.com   www.bodyforlife.com   www.bodyforlife.

*"…if I help one person feel as good as I do,
I have accomplished something important."*

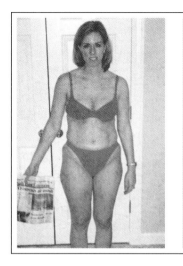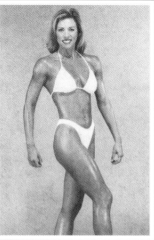

I now know what it feels like to be a winner. I know what it feels like to set your mind on a goal and accomplish it. I had no idea how much I would be changed by this experience.

When I began the Program, I was like a lot of new mothers: out of shape, tired, and uninspired. Over 16 months after my daughter was born, I still weighed 25 lbs more than before. I finally realized how bad I looked after seeing a photo a friend took of me last summer in a bathing suit. I was shocked. What happened to the young, thin, vibrant person I used to be?

I had never lifted weights before. I had never stuck to a structured nutrition plan. I was insecure and knew I would be stepping out of my "comfort zone." So, I approached the whole process with the idea of taking "baby steps" and keeping everything simple.

When I started, I weighed 148 lbs and had 29.5% bodyfat. After 12 weeks, I weighed 135 lbs with 15.5% bodyfat. And, I have lost over 20 inches! And I have never had more energy in my life. But even more empowering than my physical results is the response from family, friends, co-workers, and even strangers. No one had ever asked me for advice about how to get fit. But when others witnessed my transformation, they started asking me for help. The best part of it is I can't get through a workout without someone coming up to me and asking how I am achieving such fantastic results.

I'm sharing what I've learned with everyone I can, and if I help one person feel as good as I do, I have accomplished something important.

I have discovered that changing my physical appearance caused me to learn about my inner self. I have learned that I am determined, dedicated, strong-willed, and persistent. I also now know that I can push myself beyond physical pain and emotional blocks to achieve my goals. That is the gift this Challenge has given me, and I am eternally grateful.

Mary Queen
Age 28
Mother/Account Executive; High Point, NC

bodyforlife.com   www.bodyforlife.com   www.bodyforlife.com   www.bodyforlife.com   www.bodyforlife.com   www.bodyforlife.c

"This Challenge has taught us that ordinary people can inspire others in a way that changes lives."

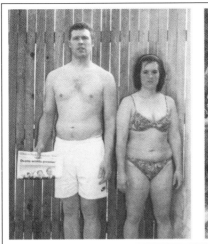 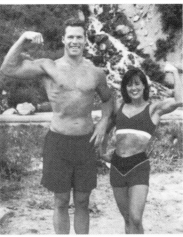

We met as college athletes. Back then, we spent hours doing cardio workouts, followed strict low-calorie diets, and had never tried weight training. We didn't realize it then, but our misconceptions about training were holding us back. Then, when we started our careers and had a son, we failed at our half-hearted attempts to keep our "college figures." For so long, we didn't know exactly what we were missing. This Challenge has given us a second chance to feel fit, energetic, and strong.

We began by planning our lives, mapping out our meals and our workouts, and writing down our goals. We juggled our schedules so we could work out and share meals together. And the adventure began.

In just a few weeks, we were looking and feeling better about ourselves. Another bonus was the money we saved giving up fast food! Family and friends started to take notice and said we not only looked fitter, we seemed happier. We were! It was less about the way we looked and more about what was happening on the inside. There were busy days, but organizing our schedule even left time for us to volunteer together with a local youth organization.

Seeing each other grow in such a positive way, so quickly, became a source of daily joy and positive energy. The ultimate triumph is realizing that we are now living at a higher level. And that has allowed us to become better parents, better at our careers, and it has also allowed us to help others transform.

This Challenge has taught us that ordinary people can share their success and inspire others in a way that changes lives. We also now know completing 12 weeks is indeed a challenge! Our secret was dedicating the tough days to others—our family and our friends, who might in some way be inspired by seeing us achieve our goals. We are devoted to helping them find the happiness we now enjoy each and every day.

Gary and Amy Arbuckle
Ages 28 and 24
Parents/Doctor and Weather Anchor; Denver, CO

Real-Life Success Stories

195

"Courage is like a muscle;
it too takes time to grow."

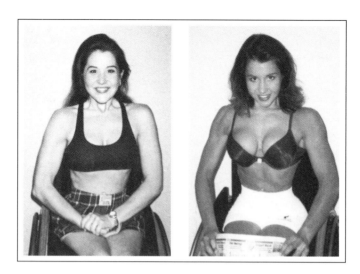

Like other people in this world, I have put many limitations on myself because of a stigma of society. Being in a wheelchair, there are many expectations of what your life should be like. For a while, I thought I was going to lead the inactive and dependent lifestyle so many people expected of me. I had built a wall around myself of embarrassment and fear.

When I learned about this challenge, a desire sparked inside of me to look forward, not back. I soon developed a passion for gaining strength. I started to have the mentality that these limits I had placed on myself for so long were no different than those that any able-bodied person has to endure in his or her own life. I have had to break beyond those self-imposed limits in order to grow in every way possible.

The main element that kept me going since I started my transformation was the idea of knowing I would have the opportunity to inspire others, to enhance both their health and their outlook on life. However, as time went on, my desire grew even more. I was starting to see tremendous improvements in my strength and my physique. I gained seven pounds of muscle, and my strength almost doubled in three months. In order for me to continue, I had to take it further and develop a deeper courage to learn, do, and succeed throughout the rest of my life.

I believe courage is like a muscle; it too takes time to grow. I believe this experience has laid the foundation for me to develop this type of courage, so I could have the power to learn, to do, to enable me to succeed. I will show others how to get beyond this first step in developing the most important "muscle": Courage.

Raven Simpson
Age 20
Student; Lubbock, Texas

196   Real-Life Success Stories

"The Challenge taught me... to make bold decisions for the right reasons and to act on them."

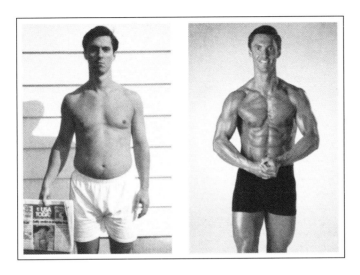

I got more out of the Challenge than I put into it. My momentum made things happen that I never expected. Family, friends, and people everywhere began to ask me what was going on. They could see the physical changes, but it was the changes in my spirit and attitude they were most curious about. I get energized sharing my story with them, answering their questions, and helping them get started with their own transformations. I could never have imagined how rewarding it would be to watch them succeed.

My mom has always given so much of herself to our family and others and never helped herself. I helped her take the first steps of this challenging and rewarding journey. And now she has succeeded beyond her wildest dreams! At age 56, she lost 15 lbs of fat while gaining muscle tone and energy in 12 weeks. She is strong and healthy, and now she inspires me. When my loved ones started to transform, their enthusiasm and success began to increase my confidence.

I've spent the past ten years working my way up to a senior position in a large pharmaceutical company. Although there were aspects of the job that were rewarding, what I realized was that my career was not fulfilling. The Challenge taught me that the only way to accomplish something meaningful was to make bold decisions for the right reasons and to act on them. So, I set new goals... and resigned.

Now, at age 32, I'm enrolled in pre-med courses. I have the confidence and sense of purpose to make my dream come true. I know I can help make a difference in people's lives.

This Challenge has made me a better person. By confronting my fear of failure and changing my habits and outlook, I have developed my character along with my body and health. By setting and committing to goals, I've learned that striving to achieve them is its own reward. By sharing my experiences and enthusiasm, I've seen how an ordinary person like me can help so many others. And, most important, I've learned that these lessons are far more valuable to me than any material prize possibly could be.

Tom Archipley
Age 32
Father/Pre-Med Student; Okemos, MI

Real-Life Success Stories

197

"I finally found my best body ever, and I'm determined to keep it!"

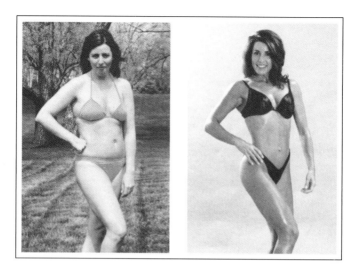

Like many women over 35, my body started to slide. I was gaining a little fat and losing some muscle tone. But, I still looked "pretty good," I thought. I didn't think I was eating wrong. And I was exercising once in a while. Then came the wake-up call. I decided to accept Bill's challenge; I weighed myself and took my "before" photo.

Yikes! I weighed over 150 pounds, and looking at that photo motivated me like I can't even explain. It was the reason—the catalyst I so desperately needed.

In the beginning, I could not tell you the difference between a barbell and a dumbbell. In fact, I couldn't even tell you where my biceps were. But as the weeks went by, I learned more and more.

The 12 weeks went fast. Before I knew it, what was once a challenge became routine. The techniques Bill taught me became a part of life. Now, I've lost 25 pounds of ugly fat and gained muscle tone and strength. I finally found my best body ever, and I'm determined to keep it!

This Program has enriched every aspect of my life, from my marriage and being a better mom and role model for our 10-year-old daughter, to my complexion. It even helped reduce my PMS symptoms. I feel as if I can do anything I set my mind to.

It's not easy juggling all the demands and pressures of working, raising a family, and completing a major transformation like this, but it's not easy living life in a body you're not comfortable with either. I commend every woman who has the strength to expose her flaws and the courage to complete the 12 weeks. I am proof that any car-pooling, kid-totin' "soccer mom" in her thirties who has lost that 20-something body *can* get it back.

Kelly Adair
Age 36
Radio Producer; Omaha, Nebraska

odyforlife.com   www.bodyforlife.com   www.bodyforlife.com   www.bodyforlife.com   www.bodyforlife.com   www.bodyforlife.co

*"My patients asked me what
I was doing to look so healthy."*

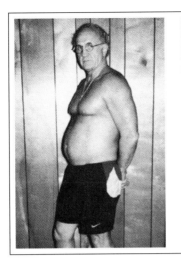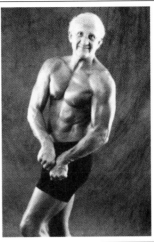

Going through a traumatic divorce left me emotionally and physically devastated, and my relationship with my daughter seemed crippled. My self-esteem had never been lower, my waist never bigger, and my cholesterol level never higher.

Then, one of my patients left a copy of Bill's magazine in my office. I was awed by the the photos. Impressed with the incredible results of others, I realized if they could do it, so could I. It was time to get control of my life.

I started exercising and set goals. The physical and emotional changes that occurred in just the first month were inspiring, and I realized my goals were achievable. I ended up reducing my body fat from 25 to 8.5 percent. My friends couldn't get over my transformation. My patients asked me what I was doing to look so healthy. More importantly, my relationship with my teenage daughter began to flourish. We even started exercising together.

My health has dramatically improved. My cholesterol went from dangerously high levels to healthy levels. My self-esteem improved, my energy level increased, and my medical practice has never been better. My life has changed as a result of this Program. I have become extremely fascinated with exercise, nutrition, and the role supplements play in improving health, fitness, and longevity. Over the next year, I intend to incorporate these anti-aging principles, along with my own experiences, into my practice.

Today I look at myself, and I feel a sense of pride. I really like what I see. I am reminded of Bob Seger's song "Lean and Solid Everywhere—Like a Rock!" Only I'm not 18 years old as he was—I'm 60!

Jeffry Life, M.D.
Age 60
Physician; Meshoppen, Pennsylvania

Real-Life Success Stories

199

"I lost 14 pounds and gained energy, muscle tone, and confidence."

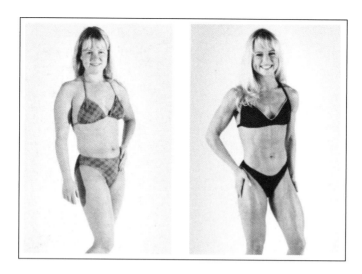

I never really truly understood until now that to feel good deep down inside, you must take care of the outside. After all, we must count on our bodies for life.

But to feel good physically, a person has to work for it, and most of us just aren't able to take that step and make that commitment. After all, don't we work enough already?

What I realized by doing this Program is that deciding what you work on—what you spend your time doing—is so important. Before, I was busy getting out of shape. Now, I'm busy getting in shape!

A true challenge is not easy. (An "easy challenge" would be a contradiction in terms.) However, the rewards and the benefits of successfully completing a true challenge far outweigh the difficult times the challenge presents.

I discovered a lot about myself, about my strengths and my weaknesses. I experienced the power of looking toward the future and promising myself I would achieve my goals. I knew what I wanted my body to look like. I visualized that body continually. And now I'm there. I lost 14 pounds and gained energy, muscle tone, and confidence.

As a result of the past 12 weeks, I've grown to enjoy exercising, and I also now understand proper nutrition. I believe the workouts not only make me look better but make me feel a lot better, too.

My life has completely turned around. I feel that I have been awakened from a 24-year-long nap. I now know much more about how strong I am, both physically and mentally. I'm creating and achieving goals in all areas of my life. I would like to share this feeling of empowerment with people. This experience has not only been a physique transformation but a life transformation as well.

Amy Yarnell
Age 24
Reno, Nevada

"I've built a stronger mind,
a stronger body, and a stronger life."

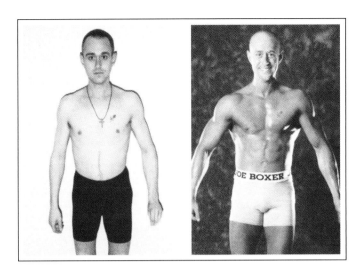

In recent years, my life seemed to be getting out of control. It felt like turbulence at 30,000 feet—you know, that feeling of being scared to death?

I was diagnosed with cancer. I was only 28 years old. It just wasn't fair. I had two choices: I could throw in the towel or believe in myself 100 percent. I decided I would live—that failure was *not* an option. (I constantly used those words for inspiration.)

Cancer is a pretty "smart disease." The type I had, called "germ-cell tumor with seminoma elements present," circulated throughout my body. It took surgeons six hours to remove 36 lymph nodes from my abdomen and chest cavity. I was confined to a hospital bed for 23 days.

I weighed only 124 pounds when I started. I followed the Program and looked forward to achieving my transformation. After 30 days, I'd already gained 10 pounds. It was already working! I was gaining confidence and feeling stronger. I ended up gaining 26 pounds of muscle. I am the talk of the Kaiserslauttern military medical community—my doctors and co-workers can hardly believe it.

I have, so far, beat this cancer. I've faced death, only to come back and be in my best shape ever. I've also gained a tremendous amount of self-confidence.

For me, it's about the accomplishments. I've built a stronger mind, a stronger body, and a stronger life.

This is just the beginning!

Michael Tate
Age 29
Medical Technician (USAF); Rammstein Air Base, Germany

Real-Life Success Stories

201